Work stress
The making of a modern epidemic

**DAVID WAINWRIGHT AND
MICHAEL CALNAN**

Open University Press
Buckingham · Philadelphia

Open University Press
Celtic Court
22 Ballmoor
Buckingham
MK 18 1XW

email: enquiries@openup.co.uk
world wide web: www. openup.co.uk

and
325 Chestnut Street
Philadelphia, PA 19106, USA

First Published 2002

A catalogue record of this book is available from the British Library

ISBN   0 335 20707 3 (pb)   0 335 20708 1 (hb)

Library of Congress Cataloging-in-Publication Data
Wainwright, David, 1965–
    Work stress : the making of a modern epidemic / David Wainwright,
Michael Calnan.
        p. cm.
    Includes bibliographical references (p.) and index.
    ISBN 0-335-20708-1 – ISBN 0-335-20707-3 (pbk.)
    1. Job stress.   2. Job stress–Great Britain.   3. Work–Psychological
aspects.   I. Calnan, Michael.   II. Title.

HF5548.85. W35 2002
158.7′2′0941–dc21   2001054895

Typeset in 10/12pt Sabon by Graphicraft Limited, Hong Kong
Printed in Great Britain by St Edmundsbury Press, Bury St Edmunds, Suffolk

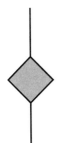

Contents

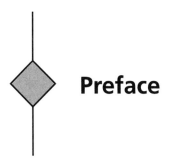

Preface

Work stress is a contradictory category; meaningful to most people living and working in western industrial societies, but at the same time the subject of ambivalence and contested claims. For many (both lay people and researchers alike), work stress indicates the 'natural' limit of human endurance and resilience, a product of the unsustainable pressures and demands placed on the worker by late capitalism; while for others the phenomenon represents nothing more than claims making by disgruntled or feckless workers backed by woolly and imprecise science.

These viewpoints may be diametrically opposed, but there is a glimmer of truth in both of them. Work stress is 'real' for many people who face problems at work. It manifests itself in *real* physical and psychological symptoms. It can have *real* consequences including behavioural change, help-seeking behaviour including clinical consultation, or even early retirement on medical grounds. Some people might benefit from their 'condition' when negotiating with employers, or, more rarely, through compensation granted by the courts, but for the majority work stress is a burden which they endure without any prospect of personal gain.

On the other hand, it is difficult to sustain the claim that work stress is simply an unmediated physiological response to 'objective' conditions in the workplace, independent of subjective interpretations and socio-cultural determinants. Is work really more demanding and pressurized than at any previous time in human history? Why was there no 'epidemic' of work stress, for instance, between the two world wars when many of those lucky enough to be in work faced incredible physical and mental hardship, uncertainty and insecurity? Why do problems and antagonisms which previously led to the picket line and the political demonstration now so often lead to the general practitioner or the counsellor? Work stress may be 'real' for those who experience it, but at the same time it is also a product of the times we live in.

This contradiction between 'realist' accounts of work stress and the more relativizing social constructionist approaches informs our approach to studying the phenomenon. Work stress is the phenomenal form taken by antagonistic production relations in western society at the current time. It is important to note that this phenomenal form is not a myth or an example of 'false consciousness' – problems at work *really are* experienced as a threat to health and well-being. However, although this phenomenon is grounded in experiences of the real world it also hides a secret. By presenting itself to consciousness in the form of an 'epidemic' with physical symptoms, an aetiology and a range of therapeutic solutions, work stress takes on the appearance of a naturalized and universal response to problems at work – as if work stress would always occur where workers face adverse experiences at work, regardless of time or place. Our aim is not to show that work stress is false, but to demonstrate that it is an historically specific and transitory phenomenon. Our strategy is to reveal the historical, structural, cultural and discursive conditions of existence that enable problems at work to be experienced through the medicalized prism of a work stress epidemic. We also explore the form of subjectivity that the work stress phenomenon gives rise to and appraise strategies for opposition or resistance.

Our analysis is grounded in qualitative study of the attitudes and beliefs of workers. We have attempted to reveal the ways in which workers make sense of their experiences at work, how they interpret and give meaning to embodied signs and symptoms, and make choices about how to respond. However, the ethnography of work stress can only get us so far because it is constituted by, as well as constitutive of, the discourse of work stress. It can tell us how people invest their experiences with meaning, but not why those explanations take the particular form of work stress. To grasp this we need to look beyond ethnographic accounts to examine the historical, structural and cultural factors that condition them. Moreover, we need to consider the public and scientific discourses on work stress to ascertain the socio-cultural influences on their production and their influence on how individuals make sense of their experiences at work.

Our epistemological standpoint means that our approach to the scientific body of evidence on work stress is twofold. While we are interested in their socio-cultural context and their discursive effects on the consciousness of workers we also view them as legitimate attempts to understand the work stress phenomenon that can provide valuable insights. Many disciplines have addressed work stress and our analysis has led us to engage critically the literature of epidemiology, psychology, physiology, social and economic history, industrial relations, psychotherapy and cultural studies. Perhaps only sociologists would be arrogant enough to attempt such a synthesis of other people's disciplines and we are sure that those working within these disciplines will find omissions and errors in our treatment of them. In our defence we can only point out that, like all interesting social phenomena, work stress does not fall neatly within disciplinary boundaries and a necessarily brief appraisal of the strengths and weaknesses of each contributing discipline is better than their complete omission. We are also mindful of Simon Williams's warning to would-be 'sociological imperialists' of the dangers of moving from having *something* to say about a topic to having *everything* to say about it. We have taken issue with some of the claims made by other disciplines, but we have also made use of their findings as a legitimate contribution to understanding the work stress phenomenon.

Given that our analysis considers the influence of socio-cultural factors on the production of knowledge about work stress by other disciplines it would be churlish to overlook the origins of our own perspective. Our epistemological and ontological assumptions can be easily divined in what follows. Most importantly, our point of departure is the active subject making sense of his or her experiences and choosing how to act within and against structural and discursive constraints and imperatives. Our 'problem' with the work stress phenomenon, and the rationale for this book, is that it brings into being a passive subject, a diminished self, and promotes a profoundly anti-humanist lowering of expectations about human potential. Rejecting the subjectivity of the work stress victim requires the development of new forms of individual and collective resistance and opposition to problems at work and the adoption of a more optimistic conception of human resilience. By providing a critique of work stress we hope to make a small contribution to that process.

Content and structure of the book

An important criticism of the scientific literature on work stress is that it tends to adopt a rather narrow concept of what constitutes 'work', defining it almost exclusively in terms of paid employment and overlooking the experiences of unpaid volunteers, home workers and carers. While we are sympathetic to such criticisms our purpose in this book is to critique the work stress phenomenon rather than expand its explanatory range; we have, therefore, limited ourselves to the scope of the existing public and scientific discourses of work stress.

Chapter 1 examines the public discourse of work stress. Evidence is presented from our analysis of public documents and media sources relating to the work stress phenomenon as it is manifest and represented in litigation, government policy, trade unionism, employers' organizations, and the media. Lay accounts and definitions of work stress are also examined using data from a qualitative study.[1] From these sources the key themes of the public discourse of work stress are derived and modelled.

In Chapter 2 scientific evidence from the disciplines of epidemiology, physiology and psychology are examined. The first half of the chapter adopts an historical approach, tracing the emergence of stress as a scientific construct and assessing the influence of social, economic and political influences on the scientific discourse. In the second half the strengths and weaknesses of the different disciplinary approaches to work stress are assessed in terms of their validity, reliability and conceptual rigour. Juxtaposition of the disciplines reveals contradictions, inconsistencies and lacunae in the different approaches.

Building on the analysis presented in the previous chapter, Chapter 3 attempts to provide a sociological basis for understanding the work stress phenomenon. Drawing on sociological approaches to embodiment and the emotions the chapter attempts to develop a theory of the self and the development of subjectivity that captures the way in which environmental, discursive and corporeal influences interact and intertwine over the life course. Unconscious processes are explored, but emphasis is placed on the role of consciousness and agency. Having established the importance of subjective meanings and definitions the chapter returns to analysis of qualitative data, this time from a case study of general practice, to see how these meanings are socially negotiated within the workplace.

Chapter 4 returns to the macro level and asks whether work has become harder or workers have become less resilient. Evidence is presented regarding changes in work, particularly job security, hours worked, intensification of effort, and new managerial techniques. The changing role of trade unions is then examined. The resilience of workers is explored by looking at cultural changes in attitudes towards emotional life, including heightened awareness of the vulnerability of bodies, the rise of victim culture and the therapeutic state. We draw together the different threads of the analysis to describe the historically specific conditions of existence of the work stress phenomenon and why it has such a powerful hold on public and scientific imaginations.

In the final chapter we examine possible responses to the work stress phenomenon. The job redesign agenda is examined and placed in its historical context before turning to the dominant response to work stress which comprises various therapeutic interventions. The medicalization thesis is examined along with criticisms of it and the Foucauldian reformulation of some of its key themes, particularly the way in which discourse gives rise to new forms of subjectivity. Qualitative data concerning lay attitudes to and experiences of formal therapeutic interventions for work stress are also examined, particularly focusing on the decision to consult, the mediating role of the doctor, and resistance to medicalization. The book concludes with a consideration of the forms of subjectivity that the work stress phenomenon brings into being and the possibility of developing oppositional identities and practices.

We have drawn from a very wide range of sources and expertise and we would like to thank all those who have made their work available and engaged in discussion with us. We would particularly like to thank Frank Furedi, Simon Williams and Francis Green. The argument presented in the book and any errors within it remain the responsibility of the authors. Finally, we would like to thank Paul Dieppe, director of the Medical Research Council's Health Services Research Collaboration, for his support and encouragement, and for ensuring that our experience of work stress was never first-hand.

 # The popular discourse

The developed world is facing a new and virulent epidemic. In Britain alone, an estimated 500,000 people believed they were affected by it in 1995,[1] contributing to the loss of between 5 and 6 million working days and costing the country more than £5 billion a year.[2] Men, women, young and old are all at risk from the epidemic, the consequences of which allegedly include anxiety, depression, ulcers, thyroid disorders, high blood pressure and heart disease.[3] Those at risk share one defining characteristic: they are all in paid employment. While work itself is not intrinsically pathogenic, the threat to health is thought to arise when the pressures and demands placed on the worker become excessive. This new epidemic is sometimes referred to as job strain, or, more commonly, as work stress.

Litigation

Public awareness of work stress has never been greater than at the current time, not least because of a number of high-profile court cases, dating from the mid-1990s, in which employees have sought compensation for health problems putatively caused by adverse experiences at work. Many such claims have been settled out of court: for example, Northumberland social worker John Walker accepted £175,000 in compensation for two nervous breakdowns which he claimed were the consequence of an unreasonable workload. Similarly, South Lanarkshire Council paid out £66,000 to Janet Ballantyne, in compensation for the stress, anxiety and depression caused by a bullying manager.

An important legal precedent was set in July 1999, when a county court awarded former town hall worker Beverley Lancaster £67,000 in compensation for a 'stress-related personal injury' caused by her employer's insistence that she relinquish her job as a draughtswoman, in favour of a more stressful position dealing with the public in a neighbourhood housing office. The ruling was the first of its kind in a British court, although the Trades Union Congress reported that 460 cases were then before the courts, and a further 7000 cases were being investigated by Unison, Mrs Lancaster's union. Commenting on the case, Unison's head of legal services claimed that

> Initially it was quite difficult to bring the case to court because people are quite dismissive of stress at work. But now employers know that if they damage the minds of their employees, they will have to pay out in the same way as if they did not repair the stairs and someone fell down and broke a leg.[4]

Following the Lancaster case, Worcester County Council offered Randy Ingram a record £203,000 in compensation, and admitted liability, for stress-related health problems stemming from his job as a warden managing travellers' sites. Mr Ingram had taken early retirement on medical grounds after encountering 'violent and abusive' behaviour from some of the travellers, and felt that he had not received adequate managerial support from his employers.[5]

In the United States (as with so many things), the work stress epidemic emerged earlier and has produced even more vivid compensation cases. Humphrey[6] describes the case of a Michigan secretary who received $7000 for the distress caused by a boss who constantly criticzed her for going to the toilet too frequently, and that of a Maine state trooper who received $5000 in compensation for the extent to which being on call 24 hours a day had adversely affected his sex life. In California workers' compensation claims for mental stress increased by 700 per cent over a ten-year period; and Humphrey notes that 'Even a judge received an award by claiming that he suffered a stroke from overwork because of an increased caseload of workers' compensation claims.'[7]

In Britain, workers seeking compensation are obliged to pursue their claims through the law courts under the Health and Safety at Work Act (1974), or the Management of Health and Safety at Work Regulations (1992). Under this system litigants are obliged to prove not only that they suffered a stress-induced illness that was demonstrably caused by conditions at work, but also that the problems were foreseeable and that their employer was negligent in failing to take preventive action.[8] In the United States the burden of proof is far lighter thanks to the no-fault workers' compensation system established a century ago. The scheme was introduced to avoid the need for litigation. Employees injured at work receive medical and lost wage benefits, but forfeit the right to sue their employers for negligence.[9] Grippa and Durbin[10] report that job stress-related claims nearly trebled between 1980 and 1986. The rapid escalation in stress-related compensation claims has created a financial crisis that threatens to bankrupt the system in some states.[11]

Government policy

High-profile court cases and the rapid escalation in compensation claims are only the most visible manifestations of the work stress epidemic. Government and trade union policies have also played a role in defining work stress as a key concern for health and safety at work. The British government's interest in health and safety at work dates back to the early nineteenth century[12] (i.e. to the Factory Acts dating from 1833), but an explicit concern with work stress has only recently emerged. Thus, following its submission to the Robens Committee[13] of 1972, the National Association for Mental Health (MIND) complained that: 'The Report has singularly overlooked the factors necessary for the promotion of mental and social well-being, as opposed to physical health and safety.'[14] Despite the Department of Employment's assurances to the contrary, the subsequent Health and Safety at Work Act (1974) failed to make explicit reference to work stress, although it did oblige employers to ensure that workplaces are safe and healthy – a general requirement, retrospectively interpreted as including an injunction to curb work stress. As late as 1992, work stress remained conspicuously absent from health and safety legislation, although the Management of Health and Safety Regulations of that year mandated employers to assess risks to health in the workplace and implement appropriate controls – which again has subsequently been taken to include work stress as a health risk.

During the 1990s the government's Health and Safety Executive (HSE) took a much greater interest in work stress, commissioning a series of research projects,[15–20] and issuing guidance and advice on stress management.[21,22] The HSE's most significant policy statement on work stress, *Stress at Work: A Guide for Employers*, was published in 1995.[23] The guidance is mainly concerned with defining work stress and suggesting management strategies for monitoring and addressing the problem. While the absence of specific legislation on work stress is noted, the guide suggests that

> . . . employers do have a legal duty to ensure that health is not placed at risk through excessive and sustained levels of stress arising from the way work is organised, the way people deal with each other at their work or from the day-to-day demands placed on their workforce. Employers should bear stress in mind when assessing possible health hazards in their workplaces, keeping an eye out for developing problems and being prepared to act if harm to health seems likely.[24]

The document goes on to claim that stress should be treated like any other health hazard. While this advice did not carry the weight of law, it did give official recognition and sanction to the problem, which may have strengthened the hand of those seeking compensation for work stress-related health problems through the law courts. Certainly, the HSE document appears to have worried employers; a survey of union health and safety representatives, commissioned by the Trades Union Congress, found that 31 per cent of employers had a policy on stress at work, 76 per cent of which had been introduced since the HSE document was published.[25] Even so, the HSE guidance is not yet legally binding, although in the face of mounting empirical evidence and persistent lobbying from the trade union movement, the Health and Safety Commission (HSC) issued a discussion document to canvass opinion on the development of a legally binding 'Approved Code of Practice' on work stress.[26] The document notes the growing body of evidence about the relationship between work stress and ill health, but is quite candid about the difficulties of effective regulation. Following the consultation exercise the HSC launched a national strategy to promote good practice, but deferred the decision to implement an Approved Code of Practice.[27]

The work stress epidemic has also influenced other strands of government policy, for example, in the pursuit of *Fairness at Work*.[28] In opposition the Labour Party pledged to reform employment law by introducing a national minimum wage; implementing the Working Time Directive's rights to paid annual leave and limits on working time; signing the Social Chapter, and introducing a statutory right to trade union recognition.[29] These commitments have largely been met. The National Minimum Wage Act received royal assent in 1998, entitling workers aged 18–21 a minimum rate of £3.00 per hour, and £3.60 for older workers (subsequently increased to £3.60, and £4.20 respectively, from October 2002).[30-1] Working time regulations also came into force in 1998, limiting to 48 the average number of hours a week that most workers can be required to work (though workers may work longer hours if they choose to). Other individual and collective employment rights (including union recognition) were recognized in the Treaty of Amsterdam, and the Employment Relations Act 1999.

Although work stress was not cited as a rationale for the employment reforms, the intention was at least partially to redress the imbalance between the interests of workers and employers that was perceived to have arisen during the 1980s. However, as Tony Blair indicated in his introduction to the *Fairness at Work* White Paper, the extent of this reversal would be limited:

> There will be no going back. The days of strikes without ballots, mass picketing, closed shops and secondary action are over. Even after the changes we propose, Britain will have the most lightly regulated labour market of any leading economy in the world.[32]

The new government's health policy was also influenced by the work stress debate. The Acheson report on inequalities in health[33] cited empirical evidence of the relationship between job strain and coronary heart disease, musculoskeletal disorders, mental illness, and sick leave, and made three rather general recommendations about improving the quality of jobs, encouraging good management practice and assessing the impact of employment policies on health. The following year, Acheson's recommendations were reflected in the government's public health strategy, which observed that 'Stress can harm people's physical health. Evidence has shown that working in jobs which make very high demands, or in which people have little or no control, increases the risk of coronary heart disease and of premature death.'[34] The Department of Health is also collaborating with the Health and Safety Executive, trade unions and employers on a 'Healthy Workplace Initiative', to ensure that staff are 'healthier, happier and here'.[35]

Despite the recent flurry of government policy, the Health and Safety Executive inspectorate remains under-resourced – on average, companies can expect a visit from the HSE inspectors once every seventeen years.[36] Added to this, the HSE's guidance on enforcement (for its own inspectors) reveals a reluctance to take action against employers who contravene work stress regulations:

> In all cases it is important not to raise expectations or give the impression that enforcement action will be taken. Attention can be drawn to the difficulty of setting and enforcing specific standards in this area . . . there is no basis for setting specific standards nor, except in exceptional circumstances, in taking formal enforcement action . . .[37]

The trade union response

With 200,000 health and safety representatives nationwide,[38] the trade union movement has stepped into the breach left by the HSE, and has taken a leading role in raising awareness of the work stress epidemic among workers and employers. Following its own survey of 7000 safety reps, which identified work stress as the main health and safety issue in British workplaces, the Trades Union Congress launched a major campaign, backed by a 'Charter on Stress', to address what it described as 'the new industrial epidemic'.[39] As well as demanding action on work stress from employers, the government, the European Commission and the HSE/C, the charter also committed the TUC to providing courses on preventing work stress and negotiating workplace agreements for union safety reps, the production of leaflets on stress for union members, and bargaining briefs to enable union negotiators to secure agreements with employers. The guidelines also demanded employer recognition of work stress, stress audits to measure prevalence, job redesign, action on bullying and harassment, counselling and support for workers suffering from work stress, and compensation where appropriate.

Many individual unions have also launched campaigns against work stress, and have encouraged their representatives to negotiate work stress policies with employers.[40] Such agreements often include recognition of the work stress problem by employers, and acknowledgement that the employer's obligation, under existing health and safety legislation (to safeguard the health of their employees and assess potential risks to health), includes psychological health. A commitment to tackling the causes of work stress, as well as providing counselling and support to sufferers, is also often included.[41–2]

The unions have also been prolific auditors of work stress, conducting surveys within particular companies or across whole industries. As well as finding very high rates of prevalence (often in excess of 50 per cent of the workforce), such surveys also increase workers' awareness of the work stress epidemic, a message backed up in leaflets, posters and branch meetings. See Chapter 4 for an historical account of how the emphasis on health and safety fits in with the changing role of the unions.

The employers' perspective

The response from employers has often been ambivalent and equivocal. A survey of 500 members of the Institute of Directors found that 40 per cent regarded stress as a big problem for their organization.[43] And the Institute of Personnel and Development has warned employers that unless they address the work stress phenomenon, they are likely to suffer increasingly high costs from litigation and loss of productivity from low morale and sickness absence.[44] Such threats are taken seriously by employers, but at the same time many are reluctant to accept the work stress epidemic at face value. The CBI's response to the HSC's discussion document (which examined the possibility of implementing an Accepted Code of Practice on work stress) captures the employers' dilemma.[45] On one hand the CBI recognizes that work stress is a legitimate health and safety issue, but quibbles with the way in which it has been conceptualized, seeing it as an individual problem stemming from variations in 'susceptibility to pressure', and pointing to the difficulty of separating out the effects of 'work and home pressures'. The CBI objected to the HSC's proposed code of practice because they felt that it was unworkable, and that it would lead to further litigation. Employers have been equally tentative in their practical efforts to address work stress, tending to focus on the provision of counselling and coercive policies for 'managing' sick leave, rather than on more radical preventative measures, such as job redesign.[46–7]

The media

The print and broadcast media have given extensive coverage of the work stress epidemic, in news items, health features, and drama. The recent compensation cases have generated a number of newspaper headlines, for instance: 'Race to cash in on the stress bonanza';[48] 'The £67,000 award that sends shivers down every boss's spine'.[49] Other aspects of the epidemic have also received attention, including the allegedly adverse effects of information technology – 'Cyber-stress panic strikes',[50] the apparent link between stress and violence at work –'Rising stress brings "desk rage" at work',[51] and the provision of telephone counselling – 'Helpline opens for stressed teachers'.[52] Reporting of the stress epidemic has also been backed up, in the colour supplements and glossy magazines, with advice on diagnosing work stress and treating it, usually with relaxation or stress management techniques. Similar themes have featured in television health and lifestyle programmes.

Television drama and comedy has also focused on the pressures and strains of modern work. During the 1970s, 'executive' stress and the desire to escape the 'rat race' was a common theme, for instance in the BBC's *Fall and Rise of Reginald Perrin* and *The Good Life*. More recently, several television dramas have attempted to take a more serious look at stress, particularly among the emergency services and health workers generally. The American television series *NYPD Blue* featured two police officers (Sopowicz and Diana) driven to alcoholism by the pressures of work, and similar themes have been explored in *The Bill* and *Cracker*. Coping (and failing to cope) with the stresses of working in the health sector are constant themes of British and American television series, such as, *Casualty, Peak Practice*, and *ER*.

Hollywood movies have pursued a similar trajectory, moving from 'executive stress' movies such as *The Apartment*, in which Jack Lemmon suffers from the stress of mundane work and intrusive/coercive management, through to more contemporary accounts of work stress among junior white-collar workers, for example *Clockwatchers*, which examines the marginalization and job insecurity of the office 'temp', and *Office Space* which juxtaposes an office worker's response to corporate downsizing with the work stress encountered by his waitress girlfriend.

Representations of work stress in contemporary popular culture may be sensationalized or superficial, but they play an important role in promoting public awareness of the epidemic, and shaping the ways in which it is perceived. A key aspect is the moral framework within which the work stress 'victim' is located. In the tradition of the 'Hollywood hero', characters who had extremely stressful experiences at work, but demonstrated their ability to cope unflinchingly with the pressure, tended to be represented in a positive light, as strong-willed resilient individuals in the John Wayne mould. And those who were not able to meet the challenge were dismissed as weak or cowardly. However, more recently the boundaries of heroism have been broadened to include a more open account of the hero *struggling* to cope; for instance, in *Star Trek: The Next Generation*, Captain Picard is able to call upon the therapeutic skills of Counsellor Troy to help him cope with the pressures of starship command – a service his predecessor Captain Kirk never needed to rely on.

Similarly, characters such as Reginald Perrin who escape the pressures of work are also presented in a positive light, because they are seen to be striving for a more meaningful, or less alienated, existence. Even those who succumb to job strain and have a mental breakdown or a heart attack may be presented, if not positively then at least neutrally, as the victims of forces beyond their control. For example, the medical drama *Casualty* has portrayed a hospital manager who had a nervous breakdown because of the stress caused by having to implement financial austerity measures, and, more recently, a bank manager who suffered a heart attack for similar reasons. Neither character was portrayed negatively; in fact, the lapse into illness was presented almost as a protest against unreasonable demands or pressure.

In contemporary drama, the only time that victims of work stress are likely to be portrayed in a morally negative way is when their subsequent behaviour becomes anti-social; for instance, a story line in the crime series *Cracker* involved police officer Beck witnessing the on-duty murder of his superior, and subsequently raping a colleague, before taking his own life. Even here, there was a degree of moral ambiguity about who was to blame for Beck's actions.

As well as promoting public awareness of the work stress epidemic, media accounts also reflect ambiguity about the moral status of the work stress victim. Those who win compensation for work stress can be presented as the unwitting victims of unreasonable demands,[53] but they may also be portrayed as examples of the 'compensation culture',[54] the implication being that their actions betray, if not opportunism, then at least an exaggerated fragility. Fictional accounts of work stress are equally uncertain, with traditional representations of heroism and weakness being frequently questioned and revised. As we shall see, this ambiguity lies at the heart of the work stress debate.

The lay experience of work stress

The above analysis is based on documentary evidence of the way in which the work stress phenomenon is represented in public discourse, but what impact do such popular representations have on people's lived experience? This question is addressed below by presenting evidence from a small qualitative study conducted among workers in the Dover locality. Twenty informants were selected from the respondents to an earlier postal questionnaire. All had reported high levels of work stress and some had consulted their general practitioner regarding this. A more detailed account of the research methodology is given in the Appendix.

We began by asking the informants which aspects of their work they found stressful. A number of themes emerged from the data, including workload, pressure, surveillance, and job insecurity. Many of these factors were presented as if they had only recently become problematic. Comparisons were often made between 'now' and the 'old days', with the implication that experiences at work had taken a sudden turn for the worse. It is perhaps unwise to accept subjective assessments of this kind at face value, as they might simply reflect a tendency to view the recent past in an overly favourable light; to construct the myth of a 'golden age' of employment, when jobs were secure and well paid, workload was light and fulfilling, and managers were supportive and helpful. The history of industrial relations in Britain suggests that this idealized image does not adequately grasp the experiences of earlier generations of workers (see Chapter 4). However, the perception of a deterioration in working conditions cannot be entirely dismissed as a romanticization of earlier experiences. Many informants referred to specific instances of managerial change that, for instance, increased their workload or reduced their job security. Not only this, but the process of managerial change in itself was often experienced as problematic, because of the extent to which it disrupted established patterns of working.

Managerial change

The privatization of publicly owned utilities and services is perhaps the most striking example of managerial change. However, similar themes emerged with reference to the merger of two companies, the transition of 'contracted out' local authority services from one private company to another, and the introduction of managerialism into the public sector. The overwhelming perception among the respondents was that managerial change was accompanied by adverse experiences for the workforce. A common complaint was that new managerial arrangements often entailed job losses, which also had adverse consequences for those who remained in employment. The following quotation comes from an informant who had retired on medical grounds from a privatized electricity utility:

> In the olden days it used to be a good laugh and we used to have good times, but since privatization it's just been cut, cut, cut, the number of staffing levels. And every year they were getting rid of about four or five project managers or engineers as you call them. All the time it's cut. There was no newcomers. There were no apprentices coming in, also they had this brilliant idea that contractors were best, and looking after contractors is sometimes more stressful than looking after your own men.

A similar point was made by a cook working at a school where catering had recently passed from one private contractor to another:

[...] this company took over about eighteen months ago and it's a typical private company; they want to make as much money as they can although they say profit making is not the main concern, but at the end of the day it is. I have cut down on the staff in my kitchen and the idea is they want me to do the same work with less staff.

As well as concerns about job losses and increased workload, informants were also worried that cost-cutting and downsizing might impede their ability to deliver high-quality goods and services. This was often expressed in terms of the long-term interests of the organization being sacrificed for short-term gain. However, this was not exclusively to do with the pursuit of profit, as illustrated by the following quotation from an NHS nurse (who had taken early retirement on medical grounds):

I think in the end it was the speed of the changes and the extra workload we were expected to take on, with very little support from the managers, for the work we were doing that they had previously done. And we were also, of course, taking on tasks that we did on the doctors' 'New Deal' with very little training and no extra support put in on the wards. So you felt very torn between care of the patient and your administrative managerial work. So we were torn between the two roles really.

The above quotation illustrates the difficulty of adapting to the new working conditions and role expectations that often accompany the process of managerial change. A further aspect of this theme is the tendency for managerial change to drive out informal and personal working relations in favour of a much more structured and 'dehumanized' regime. As the following quotation illustrates, this could leave workers feeling like a 'resource' rather than a valued employee:

[...] we don't have a personnel department now. With personnel, that word was derived from person, now it's the human resources department, you are a resource that's used.

The dehumanization of working relations also means that managerial change may be introduced in a way which fragments solidarity among workers and reduces their capacity to provide mutual support. One inform-ant who was working as a chef on a cross-channel ferry at the time of the interview had previously worked as a coal miner. When asked what he missed most about his old job, he referred to the extent to which new forms of job tenure had undermined solidarity at work:

[. . .] well, the comradeship. There's nothing like that on the ships. I don't know, they're just a different breed. It's different really. The youngsters are just ready to stab you in the back, anything just to get your job. You see I'm what they call core crew. I'm contracted and these are all temps coming in. If you've got a crew job they want your job and they'll do anything to get it.

As the above quotation suggests, terms and conditions of employment are often safeguarded for workers who were employed before the implementation of managerial change, while new employees are offered less favourable contracts. The disparity between the two groups of workers can lead to a loss of solidarity which may impede working relations, reduce mutual social support (both in the workplace and in recreational activity after work), and generally lead to a more antagonistic working environment.

Relations at work may also be damaged by structural reorganization, particularly when this entails a reduction of middle management or fragmentation of long-established support networks:

Well in the end we became so remote that we didn't have a manager in the area. My manager, when I worked in Canterbury, was at Crawley. So you're more on your own. You've got no back-up to help you. They also divided us into little networks in the district of Canterbury and we weren't allowed to help each other like we used to in the old days. If we had a fault or cable damage everybody used to be hands on and went and got it back on, but because these little cells were set up it was only part [of the organisation] that were allowed to go and I wasn't allowed to help or anything like that. And they weren't allowed to help me if I got problems. So there was a lack of support really because they were trying to set up these little cells and have their own costs and expenses, and it all boiled down to pounds, shillings and pence.

It is important to note that it is not just the consequences of managerial change that can cause problems for employees, but the process itself – the tensions and pressures of transition and their impact on organic interpersonal relations and solidarity. Superficially, this might be interpreted as an argument in favour of preserving the status quo or for assuming that the difficulties associated with managerial change will subside over time, as workers adjust to the new arrangements and develop new networks of support and solidarity. However, although the data suggest that the process of managerial change is widely experienced as problematic in itself, this perception cannot be adequately explained without consideration of the content of change, the interests served by it, and who has control over the implementation of change. These issues emerge when we consider the consequences of managerial change, the first of which concerns workload.

Workload

A heavy and unrelenting workload has long been a characteristic of certain types of blue-collar employment. Apart from the reference to the 'designer label' the following quotation from a sewing machinist in a clothing factory would be familiar to generations of textile workers:

> [...] it's a designer label so quality control is uppermost and it is not nice if you are struggling with a waist-band or something that just doesn't want to go right, you have got a little lady sitting at the end of the line saying 'Do this again.' It can be stressful then, and time, doing so many per hour, you know you've got to turn out like 57 pairs of trousers at the end of the day, and you've done about 37 and you think, you know, Where is this other 20 coming from?

Even so, many informants reported a significant increase in workload, often stemming from staff cuts. In order to cope with the burden of extra workload, some informants worked long hours (often unpaid), others were not able to take meal breaks or utilize their leave entitlement. Reports of increased workload were not restricted to workers in the private sector, nor were they exclusively the product of reduced staffing. In the following quotation a schoolteacher describes the way that paperwork encroached on her home life:

> There's a terrific amount of paperwork now. We have to justify everything we do, every little thing and that is very difficult, because when you're trying to run teams and you're doing extra-curricular activities both at lunch times and after school, you then have to go home in the evening and sit down and do paperwork as well.

A common theme of the different references to workload was that it had increased beyond a reasonable level; that it could only be managed by blurring the distinction between home and work, either by staying at work longer or by taking work home in the evenings and at weekends. In this sense workload was perceived to be a significant problem by many informants, something that was not in their best interests and over which they had very little control.

Pressure

Closely related to workload is the theme of pressure. Pressure is not just about the amount of work that an individual is presented with, but the urgency with which that work must be completed. It may also involve the difficulties of reconciling competing demands, particularly if they require the rapid acquisition of new skills. An NHS nurse discussed the role conflict she had experienced when she was asked to combine managerial responsibilities with patient care:

> I felt very pressurized by time to get things done. I mean there were monthly figures that had to be in by certain dates in addition to normally doing the off-duty and things like that, and seeing to rotas and arranging clinical care, which you're expected to do as a ward sister. We then had things that somebody else had done previously, so we had devolved to us the care of the staff, so we had all the personnel work to do with the staff, which we hadn't previously had to do. There was budgetary control which we hadn't previously had.

The informant quoted above went on to describe the way in which her commitment to patient care meant that her managerial work had to be completed at home, often causing her to work late into the night, or during holidays. This blurring of the distinction between home and work can make it difficult for workers to 'switch off' or unwind from the pressures of their job. One informant described the ways in which work was constantly intruding into his home life, with meetings called outside office hours, phone calls to his house, and even the forwarding of work to his home address:

> One thing that I disagreed with was that they were actually sending my work to my house. It didn't matter if I was on holiday or what I was doing, I always had it in my front door. In the end it got so bad that if I was on holiday I used to take them out of the front door and stick them in the boot of the company car and say I wouldn't open them until I went back to work, because if you start opening them when you're on holiday and things like that the stress is there all the time. Yet I still had a depot in Canterbury where they could have sent it to, but they insisted on sending it to your house, which I think is wrong.

It is important to note that there is nothing intrinsically wrong with occasionally working from home. Home working can provide a refuge from the interruptions and disturbances of office life. The issue is essentially one of control. There is a difference between having the flexibility to work from home occasionally and the necessity of working into the evening to cope with excessive workload or the pressure of short deadlines. In the latter case, rather than being a refuge from work, the home can be transformed into an extension of the workplace, with all the concomitant pressures. This is particularly the case where work-related mail and telephone calls are directed to the home address, generating a sense of being permanently 'on call'.

A further source of pressure is the requirement to meet high-performance criteria or quality standards over long periods of time, without adequate breaks or respite. This is a particular problem in the service sector, where workers are required constantly to present a positive image to members of the public. The following quotation comes from a steward on a cross-channel ferry:

> It's constant pressure all of the time. You've got to perform to a certain level, no matter how tired you are, how many nasty horrible people you get. You have got to have that front on all the time, and it is very hard to smile at somebody when they are shouting at you or while they're being awkward; or just downright arseholes.

Again, it is important to emphasize that the problem does not appear to be one of working to high standards, but of the fatigue that is experienced when such work is unremitting. In some occupations failure to perform to high standards can literally have life-threatening consequences either for the worker or for people to whom he or she has a duty of care. Where workload is high and the pressure to perform is unremitting, workers may experience performance anxiety, caused by the fear of making a mistake.

A key aspect of work pressure is managerial supervision, which is often the mechanism through which other pressures are brought to bear. Managerial supervision can be a useful source of guidance and instruction, as well as a means of sharing responsibility. However, many informants experienced it as a coercive force which diminished their personal discretion and control over work:

> Pressure from management; in my line of work you have constantly got people telling you how to do the job, you have got to do it that much better and spend that much less money, and you are constantly thinking about that, which I suppose is a form of stress, you know, I would call it pressure.

As with workload, pressure need not be a problem. The requirement to meet deadlines and produce work to a high standard can be very stimulating and make a positive contribution to job satisfaction and personal fulfilment. Pressure only becomes problematic when it reaches a certain level of intensity; the point at which a stimulating and challenging job becomes an onerous burden. This point of transition is in many respects a subjective affair, dependent on the individual's assessment of his or her circumstances, but the underlying factors that influence this assessment appear to be related to coercion and control. Putting oneself under pressure, freely choosing to push oneself to achieve a desired goal, is quite different to the experiences described above, where informants often found themselves coerced into an intense work rate and denied control over their productive activity. Pressure of this kind is often experienced via the mechanism of managerial supervision, which leads into the next theme: 'surveillance'.

Surveillance

Direct surveillance by management has long been part of the work experience of some blue-collar workers, particularly in the factory sector, where the supervisor or 'overseer' traditionally ensured that workers were not slacking or neglecting their work. One informant combined full-time study with an evening job as a cleaner for a large private company, where this traditional form of surveillance was practised:

> They were on your back all the time, putting pressure on you to do it better and better and better. And they never told you when you were doing well, only when you weren't doing well and when they wanted you to do more. If you did too well they gave you even more to do.

As well as maintaining productivity, surveillance of this kind also serves a disciplinary function, reinforcing a hierarchy of command and deference, which may generate resentment and ill-feeling. The following quotation comes from a steward on a cross-channel ferry:

> It makes me bloody angry to be honest with you. They [managers] walk past a piece of paper on the floor and they will walk halfway down the ship and come and say to you that there is a piece of paper up there on the floor. And then they will walk back past it purposely to watch you pick that piece of paper up. That is just a simple little thing but obviously it goes on with bigger things as well but it is like that all of the time, sort of picky.

The above quotation also illustrates the extent to which methods of surveillance traditionally associated with factory work have permeated the service sector. These traditional methods have been complemented by more indirect forms of surveillance which can be deployed to monitor the activity of employees whose work previously lay beyond the managerial gaze. One informant worked as a market researcher for a private company conducting an ongoing passenger survey on the ferries. The nature of this kind of work makes traditional forms of surveillance difficult to deploy, and relies on a degree of trust between employee and manager. However, the informant reported that her employer had quite literally sent out 'spies' to monitor the work:

> The fact that we knew that a manager was in the field with binoculars watching us at work. I have never been accused of lying in my life and suddenly here I was in the middle of a disciplinary which later turned into dismissal for being untrustworthy and it is a tremendous shock to the system.

This incident is interesting because it reveals the extent to which working practices which previously entailed a relatively high degree of worker autonomy, trust and responsibility are increasingly being subordinated to managerial surveillance. Whether an employee is caught out by a spot check or found to be working satisfactorily is immaterial; the space between manager and worker (and the degree of latitude it conferred) has been partially closed. Even the professions have not been immune to the encroachment of managerial monitoring and surveillance. This is particularly the case among the teaching profession, where the introduction of the national curriculum and other government initiatives has reduced decision latitude, and periodic assessment by the Office for Standards in Education (Ofsted) has generated new anxieties. One informant reported her experiences of 'Ofsted week':

> We were told in May the previous year and every single piece of paperwork was pulled to pieces, reviewed, revised, updated, typed up [. . .] That whole week for everybody was a nightmare. They popped into your lessons. They wrote a crit for you which in actual fact in our case we didn't get to see, the head teacher got to see, and you didn't know if you were going to be summoned because you'd done a good lesson, or summoned because you'd done a bad lesson, or just not told anything because you were in that middle band that was fine. That was incredibly stressful, and it was also backing each other up and supporting other staff who were finding it uncomfortable. And I think that's an unnecessary stress put on teachers.

Not all forms of managerial surveillance are presented in adversarial terms. Indeed, there is a growing tendency for surveillance to take the guise of pastoral care: for instance, one informant mentioned attending three-monthly 'job chats' which were supposed to be an opportunity for an informal and mutually beneficial discussion with a manager, but which were often used for disciplinary ends. Another informant had experienced difficulties at work which adversely affected her health and work performance. Her manager responded by producing an action plan, ostensibly to provide support and resolve the difficulties, but the informant suspected that the real purpose was to do with surveillance:

> I think once we'd got on the action plan, it was being monitored monthly, and in a sense I felt that I was going to see somebody every month and go through it. I suppose after about two or three of these meetings I felt it wasn't a supportive 'We'll work through it together', sort of thing, 'and see what we can do.' It was more of 'I'm monitoring what you're doing' – Big Brother. And I suppose that's why on those other two occasions I felt I didn't have the support. That kind of confirmed it I suppose, and I did wonder why I was still working there and actually started to apply for other jobs elsewhere.

Surveillance has a long history, but comments from the informants discussed above suggest that the range of surveillance has been extended to include occupations and professions that previously enjoyed greater autonomy. The range of surveillance techniques has also been extended beyond the adversarial approach, to include techniques that are redolent of pastoral care. Despite this transition, surveillance was still experienced as a form of discipline, and a potential cause of stress.

Job insecurity

The threat of loss of employment, either through the termination of a fixed-term contract or through compulsory redundancy, is perceived to be an increasingly common aspect of modern working life, and several informants were aware that they could no longer expect to have a 'job for life':

> I think in my parents' day, my father was a miner and I think, not because he was a miner, I think it happened in a lot of industries, he would go in at a certain age and he could be there until he retired. That is not the case any longer, you are no, you can't consider a job for life, there is no such thing.

Several informants expressed concern about job insecurity, but did not give the impression that it was a very prominent or pressing cause of work-related stress. Perhaps this is because, unlike other problems at work, job loss can easily be put to the back of the mind until it becomes an imminent threat: 'I am the sort of person, I am quite laid back until it happens and then, my god; I will panic then, but it is no good worrying about it until it actually does happen.'

Where change was afoot, for instance in the privatization of a local authority nursing home, job insecurity also comprised anxiety about future pay and conditions, as well as fear of redundancy:

> I would say that they are worried about their jobs, I mean we are paid really well, they are worried about the wages, they are worried about whether they will get paid for sick, will they get the same amount of holidays?

One area where job insecurity was perceived to have an effect was as a means of ensuring that workers were compliant with managerial policy and decision making:

> The job insecurity I think has an awful lot to do with it because you are constantly worried; it is in the back of your mind that if you don't play the game, you could be out on your ear.

That job insecurity was not a very prominent aspect of work-related stress among the informants does not mean that it can be dismissed – in small qualitative studies of this kind absence of evidence cannot be interpreted as evidence of absence. However, it does seem reasonable to suppose that the nature of job insecurity is such that, until it becomes absolutely imminent, it is unlikely to act as a direct cause of stress during the working day even though it may be a cause of anxiety or depression at other times. Moreover, it may be (as the last quotation suggests) that the most important effect of job insecurity on work stress is indirect: reducing the worker's willingness or ability to resist other stressors like heavy workload or pressure (although see the quantitative evidence in Chapter 4).

Other problems

The themes reported above occurred frequently in the interview transcripts and appear to be the most prominent factors associated with work stress, at least among the population studied. Other factors were also reported, but less frequently, perhaps by only one or two informants; they included harassment and bullying (from managers and colleagues), working inconsistent or unsocial shifts, commuting long distances, poor working environment (especially noise and dirt), and fear of litigation from the public.

Change was a common theme in the informants' discussion of work stress. This is partly attributable to the unsettling effects of rapid change; the way in which it can disrupt long-established patterns of working and undermine supportive interpersonal relations. However, it would be wrong to conclude that work stress is an inevitable attribute of change *per se*. It may be true that workers currently view managerial change with trepidation, but this might be because such change is rarely perceived to be in their interests. The themes discussed above reveal an historically specific process of managerial change, driven by the need to raise the productivity of the workforce, either as a means of increasing profits (in the private sector) or improving efficiency (in the public sector). In this context managerial change often means job losses, and, for those that remain in work, increased workload, pressure, and job insecurity. For many workers these changes amount to a substantial reduction in the amount of control they are able to exercise over their working lives. This is particularly the case where new techniques of surveillance have reduced the scope for the exercise of personal discretion and decision latitude, in favour of increased managerial regulation.

The work stress discourse not only comprises a critique of adverse experiences at work, but also the belief that such experiences give rise to poor mental and physical health. We were interested in the extent to which this putative relationship was shared by the informants. We began by asking them about symptoms of work stress.

Symptoms

When asked how stress affected them, the informants came up with a wide range of physical, psychological and behavioural 'symptoms'. Many inform-ants blurred the distinction between these different types of symptoms, for instance by suggesting that work stress caused psychological problems which manifested themselves in physical or behavioural forms. Even so, the three categories are useful for summarizing the data, which are presented in Table 1.1 below, using the informants' descriptions rather than clinical classification:

Table 1.1   Reported symptoms of work stress

Physical	Psychological	Behavioural
Palpitations	Anxiety	Throw or kick things
Stomach trouble	Talking waffle	Poor performance at work
Loss of appetite	Panic attacks	Smoking heavily
Headaches	Mood swings	Lose temper with managers
Breathing problems	Depression	Heavy alcohol consumption
Heartburn	Anger	Irritation with family
Eczema	Mental breakdown	Inability to relax with friends
Biliousness	Attempted suicide	Reclusiveness
Sweating	Uptight	Neglect housework
Dizziness	Sleeplessness	Neglect children
Light-headedness	Lethargy	Lack of concentration at work
Irregular heartbeat	Agitation	Standards of work drop
Heart attack	Irritability	
Diarrhoea	Bad temper	
Colds	Acrophobia	
Anaemia	Agoraphobia	
Tiredness	Forgetfulness	
Irritable bowel		
Shaking		
Chest pain		
Weight loss		

It is not just the range of symptoms that is surprising, but the variation in severity. The physical symptoms range from the fairly minor physiological sensations associated with the fight or flight response: palpitations, sweating, dizziness, light-headedness, shaking, through to more severe and longer last-ing symptoms: stomach trouble, breathing problems, diarrhoea, chest pain, weight loss. Some informants referred to physical complaints that one might not expect a lay person to attribute to stress, for instance, anaemia, eczema and colds.

The reporting of psychological symptoms followed a similar pattern to the physical ones, ranging from short-term affective symptoms, like anger and irritability, through to more severe, lasting complaints, like depression, even in one case to the point of mental breakdown and attempted suicide. Again, there were symptoms that one might not immediately attribute to work stress, like acrophobia for instance:

> I used to work in Canterbury and I used to go to Canterbury West [train station] and I used to have to work up at Westgate, and the thing is, to cross that road bridge to get to the park from the city walls, the stress was so bad, all I could do was concentrate on the join in the tarmac down the centre of the footpath, for me to get across that bridge, to get down on the ground again. I felt that if I had looked at the cars I would have fallen over the fence. That is how bad the stress was.

The behavioural symptoms tended to be consequences of the psychological symptoms, for instance, strained relations with family, friends and managers, poor performance of work tasks. Others might be classed as coping responses: kicking or throwing things, increased alcohol or tobacco consumption.

Most informants who had symptoms reported a combination of physical, psychological and behavioural responses. Interestingly, some informants appeared to perceive their symptoms as a response to a vague and unspecified underlying cause that they referred to as being 'a bit stressed' or 'stressed out', for instance:

> I do suffer from eczema and when I get stressed my eczema flares up again, and it's like a warning sign that I'm getting a bit stressed, so I usually try to work out what's stressing me and deal with it before the problem gets too bad. This time I was dealing with my eczema but I couldn't deal with the stress because it was out of my hands. I wasn't in control of the problem.

This concept of 'being stressed' is an interesting one, because it appears to refer to an embodied condition that mediates between exposure to problems at work (or other external problems) and the perception of physical, psychological, or behavioural symptoms. Indeed, symptoms are reported as a 'sign' of this condition: for instance, in the above quotation eczema is a sign of being stressed, and in the following quotation the informant knows that he is 'stressed out' because of his behaviour: 'I know if I get stressed out because I blow my top. So I throw something, anything at all, kick it up the old alley way.'

Being 'stressed' appears to refer to the physiological changes that occur when an individual is exposed to stressful stimuli, and which only enter consciousness when they are experienced as physical, psychological or behavioural symptoms. This leads into the theme of causality.

Causality

It was noted above that work stress is often conceptualized as a duality; as both problems at work and their consequences for the individual, in terms of physical, psychological and behavioural symptoms. As the previous section indicated, the range of symptoms is wide and many might stem from other causes. How is it then that problems at work and symptoms of ill health come to be linked causally, and what is the character of this relationship perceived to be?

For some informants, problems at work were advanced as the only cause of their symptoms, either because the problems at work were so severe or, as the following quotation suggests, because no other potential causes were perceived to exist:

> When I first took the job on I used to come home and worry a lot. Just after I took the job on I lost a lot of weight. Nothing else in my life has changed and there is no apparent reason for me to lose this much weight, but I have and I put this down to the job, that's the only thing it can be. Certainly, in the early days I worried that I wasn't going to get things done on time, and that I had took on too much.

Some informants mentioned work stress as the primary cause of their health problems, and then went on to reveal other possible causes. For example, in the following quotation an informant who had retired on medical grounds, following a heart attack, reveals a multi-causal understanding of his problem, albeit one derived from other people:

> I was told when I had the attack that really and truly it was a combination of everything. It was smoking, it was stress at work, everything combined. They can't put their finger on something and say, 'Yes, it was triggered by that', but they say, 'It's just a build up of everything over the years', and it's knocked me out that way.

That health problems associated with experiences at work often occur in the context of other adverse 'life events' was a theme commonly reported by other informants. The assumption appeared to be that one had a reserve of mental health that adverse life events slowly depleted; when the reserve was exhausted physical or psychological ill health ensued. Problems at work were often cited as the primary cause of such problems: 'You know, you can't just put it all down to work, but work, because you are at work the best part of the time, is a major factor.'

Not only do those in full-time employment spend a substantial part of their lives at work, it may also be the place where their psychological and physical resilience is most intensively tested and where failure to perform is least likely to be tolerated. This may partly account for the explanatory primacy given to 'work' in some of the informants' theories of causality, although it should be remembered that informants were selected because they had reported high levels of work stress in the survey, and also that the focus of the interview was on work, which may also have influenced the informants.

The existence of a multi-factorial and cumulative model of causality is also suggested by 'final straw' arguments, in which a particular incident pushes the individual into ill health. In the following extract a National Health Service (NHS) nurse who had reported severe problems with workload and pressure at work, as well as other life events such as recent childbirth and her husband becoming unemployed, reports how the sudden death of a colleague in similar circumstances to herself finally caused her to break down:

> What finally triggered me into going off sick was a friend of mine who had been working in the NHS in fact died very suddenly and unexpectedly. And before we knew what she'd actually died of it just occurred to me I could be next. That, I think, made me stop and look at myself. That was on a Thursday [. . .] On the Tuesday I think I'd had time for it to catch up on me and I just couldn't go in any more. Little knowing it was going to be the last time I ever went to work.

The above quotation is interesting not just because it illustrates the way in which a particularly stressful event can act as a 'final straw', but also because it reveals the extent to which the informants' interpretation of events can influence entry to the sick role – it was not just that the death of a colleague was stressful, but that it prompted a reassessment of the informant's circumstances and led to the conclusion that 'I could be next'. That there can be an interpretive element to the pathway from problems at work to ill health should not imply that the process is under-determined or freely chosen; behaviour can be both conscious and irresistible. In any case, illness (particularly physical illness) was not always consciously opted into, nor was a conscious link with problems at work always made prior to the onset of symptoms. For instance, an informant who had taken early retirement on medical grounds, following a heart attack, described the way in which he was unaware of his health problems until the heart attack occurred, and only developed a theory of causality (which included work stress, among other factors) after the event.

This theme of work stress whittling away at an individual's physical or psychological reserves 'behind the scenes', or beneath the level of conscious awareness, was reported by other informants. Even when symptoms presented, they were not always attributed to problems at work in the first instance. Medical intervention was often the point at which a causal association with problems at work was adopted:

At first I just went for the painkillers for the headaches. The doctor didn't examine me. He didn't look any further into it. And then I had a nasal problem soon after that, and I couldn't breathe through my nose. It was like an allergy and in the end I had an operation on my nose and that was a success. And they think that was stress-related; but I didn't feel stressed – I didn't think of it as an illness [. . .] it wasn't until the end of it all that I began to realize that it's probably stress-related.

The role of the general practitioner in labelling health problems as work-related is examined at greater length in Chapter 5.

In this section we have presented evidence that, as well as comprising problems at work, work stress is also experienced by some people as physically embodied 'symptoms'. These symptoms range from relatively minor and transient conditions, like sweating, dizziness and bad temper, through to severe and long-lasting physical and psychological problems. The process by which informants came to associate their symptoms with problems at work was often not automatic or straightforward. For some, problems at work were perceived to be the only cause of their symptoms, but it was more often the case that work stress was seen as the most prominent cause among a series of other factors. A common assumption appeared to be that the individual had a reserve of well-being that could be eroded by work stress and other external factors. When this reserve became exhausted, it was felt that illness would follow. In some cases the sick role was consciously entered into as a result of an individual's interpretation of events. However, the pathway from problems at work to ill health was often largely unconscious, with theories of causality only emerging after the event, sometimes in response to prompting by the medical profession.

The discourse of work stress

The documentary evidence presented in the first part of this chapter suggests that the work stress epidemic is deeply embedded in the popular imagination as a result of high-profile court cases, government policy, trade union activity, initiatives by employers, and representations in popular culture. Moreover, evidence from the qualitative study presented above shows that many of the themes of this public discourse can also be found among workers as a means of making sense of both adverse experiences at work and the onset of illness. In both the public debate and the lay accounts, work stress is an amorphous category, often poorly defined, and capable of supporting quite different interpretations and explanations. However, despite the lack of conceptual precision, common themes and assumptions can be identified, and it is not unreasonable to claim that there is a distinct and recognizable discourse of work stress. This is not to imply a tightly sutured consensus. The Trades Union Congress (TUC) and the Confederation of British Industry (CBI), for example, have expressed quite different views on the topic, and lay accounts may be different to both. However, many such disputes are accommodated within the broad contours of the work stress discourse, and there is little evidence to suggest that more fundamental challenges have had any impact on the debate.

Figure 1.1 illustrates the key elements of the work stress discourse, based on an analysis of the documentary and qualitative evidence discussed above. Put simply, the work stress discourse comprises the belief that paid employment has changed over the last twenty years, in ways which have increased the demands placed on workers while simultaneously reducing their rights

Figure 1.1 The discourse of work stress

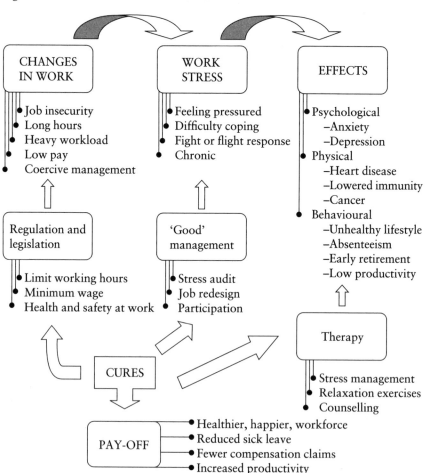

and entitlements; that these changes have led to an increase in job strain or work stress, which in turn has led to a greater prevalence of psychiatric and physical morbidity. This putatively causal series of relationships between changes in work, the experience of work stress, and negative effects on health, is the central mantra of the work stress discourse. As well as a model of the problem, the work stress discourse also comprises a series of potential solutions or 'cures', which involve intervention at each of the three points in the pathway from changes in work to health effects. The first form of intervention is aimed at reversing (or at least ameliorating) the changes in work described above, and entails regulation and legislation, such as the national minimum wage and limits on weekly working hours.

The second level of intervention concerns 'good' management in the workplace, and entails monitoring stress levels and implementing organizational changes to lessen the extent of job strain. Finally, the third level of intervention focuses on providing support or 'therapy' for the individual worker, in the hope of preventing or ameliorating the psychological, physical and behavioural effects of work stress. The assumption is that a concerted campaign of intervention, at the three levels described above, will pay off, not just in terms of improvements in the health and well-being of workers, but also through a reduction in costs to business and a significant improvement in productivity.

The purpose of this book is to demonstrate that the discourse of work stress, as it is described above, and as it is represented in the law courts, government and trade union policy and popular culture, and manifest in lay accounts of the phenomenon, is unsatisfactory. We will argue that the network of alleged relationships that comprise the discourse of work stress is derived from a selective interpretation of existing empirical evidence, and that the assumptions on which much of that empirical evidence is based are also questionable and open to reformulation. Our aim is not to deny that adverse experiences at work can ultimately lead to ill health, but to revise radically the perceived pathway between the two. Our main theme is that the 'epidemic' of work stress is really nothing of the kind – at least not in the way that epidemiologists usually define the term. These conclusions stem from a critique of key elements of the work stress discourse, which includes the following points.

Changes in work are viewed from a largely ahistorical perspective

The work stress discourse is based on the truism that paid employment is in a constant state of flux; however, two fundamental assumptions are made. First, that recent changes in the organization and experience of work are, on balance, negative, at least from the worker's perspective – greater job insecurity, longer working hours, heavier workload, lower pay, and the introduction of coercive management have all been cited as evidence of this transformation. Secondly, the beginning of this intensification and liberalization of labour is dated to a particular historical conjuncture, roughly the mid- to late 1970s. Crucially, the genealogy of changes in work is not usually traced beyond this point, and the current state of paid employment is, by implication, contrasted with a golden age of work, characterized by 'a job for life', manageable workload, adequate remuneration and sympathetic management. The following statement from the *Report of the Independent Inquiry into Inequalities in Health* exemplifies the limited historical perspective of the work stress discourse:

> For those in paid employment, there have been major changes in the nature of work stress over the past two decades. Along with greater market flexibility and deregulation of employment contracts has come greater job insecurity. Indeed, it could be considered that the concept of a secure 'job for life' is now obsolete.[55]

Locating the origins of work stress in relatively recent changes in employment is essential to the discourse of work stress, because it provides a plausible answer to the question of why the 'epidemic' emerged at this point in time. However, there are problems with such a position. The quality and security of paid employment may well have diminished over the last two decades, at least for some workers, but are conditions really worse than at any other point in history, say the 1930s for instance? If not, why are there no other documented epidemics of work stress? These issues are explored in Chapter 4.

The origins of work stress are exclusively located in changes in work, to the oversight of other social, political and cultural factors

If the work stress epidemic cannot be explained purely in terms of an historically unique high point of adverse experiences at work, then other social, political, institutional and cultural factors must also be viewed as potential antecedents of the phenomenon. Rather than assuming that work stress is exclusively an automatic response to changes in the character of paid employment, we need to consider the factors that have led adverse experiences at work to be increasingly interpreted within a psycho-medical idiom, rather than being addressed through the traditional strategies of politics and industrial relations. The erosion of solidarity in the workplace, the individuation of work, the exhaustion of socialist alternatives to the market, and the diminution of trade union power have eroded the viability of collective solutions to problems at work. And the heightened awareness of physical and mental vulnerability, coupled with the growing culture of victimhood and the therapeutic state have also encouraged workers to interpret their experiences in personal and emotional terms. Yet the possibility that the emergence of the current epidemic might be attributable to such factors does not figure prominently in the discourse of work stress. These issues are also explored in Chapter 4.

Virtually any adverse experience at work can be defined as a cause of work stress

The focus might be exclusively on adverse experiences at work as the cause of work stress, but this limitation still allows for a long list of pathogens. The qualitative evidence presented above demonstrated the wide range of problems at work that were classified as causes of stress by the informants in our relatively small study. Others have claimed an even broader range of pathogens. Table 1.2 lists the possible sources of stress in the workplace described by a recent guide for managers on how to deal with stress in higher education.[56]

To this already extensive list, the Labour Research Department[57] would add: overcrowding, badly designed furniture, poor maintenance, dangerous equipment, working with visual display units, poor childcare facilities, need for time off to care for sick dependants, machine-paced work, surveillance and monitoring, repetitive work, responsibility for others' lives, uncertain responsibilities, new technology, underuse of skills, unsympathetic management, financial constraints, rigid hierarchy and harsh disciplinary procedures.

Table 1.2 Possible sources of stress in the workplace

Physical conditions	Job design	Work organization and conditions
Noise	Inconsistent	Continual changes in work
Poor lighting	management	organization and structure
Poor temperature	Lack of support or	Lack of control over work
control	assistance	Job insecurity
Poor ventilation	Social isolation	Unclear reporting lines
Poor equipment	Poor communication	Excessive working hours
Poor workstation	Bullying	Lack of participation in decision
Exposure to fumes	Harassment	making
Exposure to the	Customer/client	Inadequate staffing
elements	complaints	Lack of recognition or promotion
	Lack of appropriate	prospects
	training	Over-promotion
	The threat of violence	Shift work
		Complexity and demands of
		new systems
		Low pay or low status
		Lack of facilities for rests or breaks
		Lone working
		Excessive workload

Essentially, any adverse experience at work, from the mild discomfort of badly designed furniture through to the trauma of a physical assault, can be defined as a cause of work-related stress. The surfeit of possible causes makes the prevention of work stress a difficult goal to achieve, particularly since some of the stressors require the achievement of a fine balance to be drawn, for example, between underutilization and overwork, or lack of promotion prospects and over-promotion. Despite such difficulties, many contributors to the work stress debate emphasize the importance of prevention, rather than 'cures' like counselling or stress management, on the reasonable grounds that prevention is better than cure. But is it really a viable or desirable project to remove from the workplace every characteristic that could be deemed a potential cause of stress? If not, what role can or should individualized therapies play? This issue is explored in Chapter 5. Scientific evidence relating to the causes of stress is examined in Chapter 2.

The allegedly causal relationship between objective conditions in the workplace and their effect on the individual is mediated by subjective factors

The difficulty lies in clarifying the precise character of the relationship between the above stressors and the experience of job strain or work stress. The discourse of work stress clearly asserts that this is a causal relationship, but is unclear about the degree of exposure required to trigger the stress response, either in terms of the type and number of stressors or the duration of exposure. It is often suggested that there is a threshold between work which is stimulating and challenging and that which is excessively demanding and, therefore, stressful. This has led some commentators to distinguish between good and bad stress, although the convention is increasingly to reserve the term for 'pressures that have harmful effects'.[58] The problem is that this threshold is not determined exclusively by objective conditions in the workplace, but by the relationship between those conditions and the resilience of the individual, as the HSE concedes:

> . . . there is no simple way of predicting what will cause harmful levels of stress. People respond to pressure in different ways. An exciting challenge to one person might be a daunting task to another; a repetitive job might be viewed by some as boring or monotonous, but others feel comfortable with routine.[59]

As the above quotation implies, there is a deeply subjective element in the pathway from objective conditions in the workplace to the experience of work stress. This would appear to throw some of the responsibility for managing work stress back on to the individual worker. The CBI has noted the difficulty of addressing work stress, when an individual's problems may stem from a combination of work and home pressures. But even in the absence of 'home pressures' there may be significant variations in resilience that are attributable to a wide range of social and cultural experiences. The trade unions have been quick to denounce this potentially 'victim blaming' approach:

> If problems at work contribute to a person's ill health, then the employer is responsible. Just because a person's asthma was caused by an out of work event does not absolve the employer from carrying out dust control measures which would alleviate the person's respiratory problems.[60]

However, the comparison with physical hazards, such as dust, is of limited value, first because the alleged causes of work stress are so many that it is difficult to imagine a workplace where all potential stressors have been controlled, and secondly, because one person's stressor may be another person's challenge – thus, even if it were viable, the removal of all the factors that could potentially cause stress to the most vulnerable worker would leave many workers feeling that their jobs had been rendered bland and unchallenging.

An alternative strategy to eradicating all potential stressors from the workplace is to ensure that individual workers are only exposed to a degree of stress that they personally are capable of dealing with, although, as we shall see, this strategy may have unintended negative consequences. These issues are addressed in Chapters 2 and 5.

The stress response is poorly specified, and the role of consciousness in its operation tends to be overlooked

Moving on from the causes of work stress, the second aspect of the discourse concerns the actual condition of work stress or job strain as it is experienced by the individual, in response to the stressors described above. This is often described as 'feeling under pressure', or having difficulty coping. Some accounts refer to the 'fight or flight' response – the physiological changes that occur in the body in response to a perceived threat. These changes are usually short-lived and are not usually seen as a threat to health, as the body rapidly returns to 'normal' as the perceived threat recedes. Problems arise when the individual feels constantly threatened, or constantly under pressure, and the physiological changes are sustained over a long period of time. It is this chronic form of stress that is believed to lead to psychological and physical illness, and to have a negative effect on performance and behaviour.

The fight or flight response is a relatively precise condition that can be measured with physiological tests (see Chapter 2), but there is a question about how closely this condition fits with the more general usage of the term work stress. Those who claim to be suffering from work stress may be referring to any one of a number of different emotional states, including low morale, frustration, feeling under-valued, low self-esteem, guilt, dis-satisfaction, or disillusionment. These are all negative emotions that may affect an individual's social functioning and job performance, but does unhappiness of this kind necessarily activate the more specific fight or flight response, and if not, is it really a health issue? The discourse on work stress tends to finesse this question by blurring the distinction between the fight or flight response and other emotional states that might result from adverse experiences at work. But this distinction is crucial when it comes to obtaining accurate estimates of the prevalence of work stress, particularly those which rely on self-reported data. When workers report that they are suffering from job stress, do they mean that they are constantly experiencing the fight or flight response, or simply that they are unhappy in their work?

A second problem relates to the way in which the fight or flight response is conceived. It is commonly claimed that stress is an occupational injury that should be viewed in the same way as a physical injury, and the implica-tion is that the fight or flight response is simply an unconscious physiological response triggered by an external stimulus, in the same way that a scab forms over a wound, without the mediation of human consciousness (although scab formation is usually associated with healing, whereas prolonged activation of the sympathetic nervous system is considered injurious). But even uncon-scious physiological responses like the fight or flight response may, over the life course, be mediated by conscious appraisals, as the body learns to unconsciously recognize particular external conditions as a threat. Leav-ing aside innate predispositions, there must be social reasons why some individuals experience a particular set of work characteristics as an anxiety-inducing threat, whereas others find the same circumstances to be a stimulat-ing challenge. We have already noted that a broad range of social, political, institutional and cultural factors may account for these variations, and that our collective or aggregate resilience may vary historically. Thus, the rela-tionship between adverse experiences at work and activation of the fight or flight response is qualitatively different to, say, exposure to a physically harmful substance like asbestos, and the onset of physical health problems like asbestosis. In the former instance, the relationship between cause and effect is mediated by the consciousness of the individual, whereas in the latter case, the injury is caused irrespective of the beliefs and perceptions of the worker. These issues are explored in Chapters 2 and 3.

Work stress has multiple health effects, each of which has multiple causes

As with the causes of work stress, the alleged effects on health and behavi-our are extensive. Table 1.1 listed the range of symptoms identified in our small qualitative study; Table 1.3 lists the 'stress symptoms' identified by the Labour Research Department.[61]

Table 1.3 Health and behavioural effects of work stress

Physical symptoms	Mental health symptoms	Social symptoms
Headaches and migraine	Irritability	Heavy drinking, smoking
Raised cholesterol	Withdrawal	or use of drugs
Digestive tract disorders	'Burn out'	Increased accident rates
Thyroid disorders	Depression	Eating disorders
Pregnancy problems	Anxiety	Relationship breakdown
Colds and other	Post-traumatic stress	Increased sickness absence
respiratory infections	disorder	
Increased blood pressure	Suicide risk	
Heart disease	Low self-esteem	
Diabetes		
Sleepless nights		
Asthma		
Ulcers		
Increased cancer risk		
Menstrual disorders		
Lethargy		

Leaving aside, for a moment, the question of whether the allegedly causal relationship between work stress and the above health and behavioural problems is supported by empirical evidence, it is important to note that the aetiology of all the alleged effects of work stress is multi-causal: for example, heart disease, depression, and relationship breakdown may be caused by a wide range of factors, independently of the effect of work stress. This in itself does not refute the claim that work stress is a contributory factor, but it does cause particular problems for the epidemiologist who tries to demonstrate the link. These problems will be examined in Chapter 2; for now it is sufficient to note that the work stress epidemic is quite different to other epidemics, in that it comprises an allegedly causal relationship between an extremely wide range of putative pathogens and an equally diverse range of health and behavioural effects, and that this relationship is primarily mediated by consciousness.

The proposed 'cures' for work stress amount to a lowering of expectations regarding human resilience, and are based upon the assumption of a passive subject, rather than an active social agent

The discourse of work stress not only comprises an account of the relationship between working conditions and ill health, but also a range of potential 'cures'. The proposed 'cures' include regulations and legislation to reverse or at least limit the harmful effects of recent changes in work; encouraging 'good' management to reduce job strain, and the provision of therapy to meet the needs of those suffering from the effects of work stress.

In their own right many of these measures may benefit workers. For example, government legislation to ensure a minimum wage, or limit the number of hours that workers can be obliged to work by their employers, or give a statutory entitlement to unpaid paternity leave, may all be welcomed by workers as a means of reducing the burden of work. Similarly, if managers strive to enrich the quality of jobs and involve workers in decision making, this can hardly be viewed as intrinsically wrong, nor can the willingness to provide psychotherapeutic support to those who feel that they need it (if its effectiveness can be proved).

The question is whether such measures constitute genuine 'cures' for work stress, and what effect their articulation as such may have on the consciousness and resilience of the worker. The problem arises because, as we have suggested, there is both a socio-cultural and conscious dimension to the work stress epidemic. Essentially, our thesis is that the work stress epidemic represents an individualized and historically specific response to adverse experiences at work, in which workers come to internalize their problems as emotional or health issues due to a diminished expectation of both their resilience and agency.

Rather than challenging these low expectations, the prescribed 'cures' for work stress may well accentuate the worker's sense of vulnerability, frailty and powerlessness, by reinforcing the belief that work is inherently hazardous, and that we need to reduce our expectations of what workers can reasonably be expected to withstand or achieve. Therapeutic intervention is based on the assumption of a passive subject, who needs to be acted upon, for his or her own benefit or protection, rather than on the conception of a resilient, active agent of change. While such measures may well bring a short-term amelioration of the symptoms of work stress, their long-term efficacy is more questionable. If the work stress epidemic is largely the product of an historically specific tendency to conceptualize adverse experiences at work in terms of emotional distress and ill health, then measures which reinforce perceptions of human frailty and passivity are unlikely to provide a lasting solution, and may even lead to an escalation of the phenomenon.

In this chapter we have examined the discourse of work stress as it appears in public institutions like the law courts, government and trade union policy, and the media. We have also attempted to illustrate the extent to which themes from the public discourse of work stress are used by workers to make sense of their experiences. The role played by scientific inquiry and empirical evidence in supporting this discourse has been deliberately omitted, and is addressed in Chapter 2 where the emergence of work stress in the disciplines of epidemiology, psychology and physiology is examined and quantitative empirical evidence is brought to bear on the problems of the work stress discourse described above.

2 The scientific construct

Work stress is deeply embedded in the public imagination. High-profile court cases, the activities of government agencies and trade unions, and representations in the news media and popular culture have combined to provide an explanatory framework through which adverse experiences at work may be filtered. This popular discourse of work stress is often couched in quasi-scientific terms, drawing much of its legitimacy from implicit and explicit references to a body of empirical and theoretical work, but what is the relationship between scientific and popular accounts of the phenomenon? Does the scientific evidence support the truth claims of the public discourse? And to what extent is the scientific discourse of work stress influenced by the social, cultural and political context in which it is produced?

The above questions are addressed in this chapter, first by examining the historical development of work stress as a scientific category, revealing the revisions and shifts in emphasis that have occurred over time, not just in response to the accretion of evidence, but also as a result of the changing social and political climate. The analysis then turns to a more detailed account of the contributions different scientific disciplines have made to our understanding of work stress, starting with epidemiological accounts of the relationship between work characteristics and health, moving on to biological evidence of the physiological changes that occur in the stressed body, and concluding with an examination of psychological insights into the factors that mediate the pathway from experiences at work to the onset of illness. The chapter concludes with an assessment of whether the public discourse of work stress is supported by the scientific evidence, and an appraisal of the inconsistencies, weaknesses and limitations of that scientific knowledge.

A brief history of stress

Despite its ubiquitous usage, 'stress' has a relatively brief history as a means of describing a psychological state. Textbook accounts often trace the genealogy of stress back to the work of Walter Cannon,[1-2] or Hans Selye.[3-7] Cannon was writing about 'emotional stress' as early as 1914,[8] but his use of the term was fundamentally different to the psycho-social category employed today. Similarly, despite his own claims to the contrary,[9] Selye's early research not only overlooked the social and psychological dimension, but omitted to use the word stress at all. In fact, psycho-social stress was not widely accepted into the scientific lexicon until after the Second World War, even though, as Newton et al.[10] note, many writers[11] have sought to extend the genealogy of the stress discourse by annexing what is in fact a prehistory of the category in use today. Despite this apparent revisionism, Cannon and Selye have had a fundamental influence on the subsequent development of the stress discourse and it is worth pausing to examine not only the content of their work, but also the intellectual climate that gave rise to it.

The prehistory of stress coincided with the ascendancy of social Darwinism and the eugenics movement. Darwin[12-13] described human evolution in terms of constant physiological adaptation to a hostile and changing environment. Nature gave rise to small incremental changes (mutations) in the organism and those which were of adaptive value conferred reproductive advantages, ensuring natural selection or 'survival of the fittest'. The social Darwinists took the theory of evolution as a template for explaining social relations, suggesting that inequalities in wealth and power were an unavoidable product of natural selection. Another central concept in the social Darwinist world view was the dominant role ascribed to instinct as a determinant of human behaviour. In 1914 Graham Wallas published *The Great Society*[14] in which he suggested modern society failed to provide an appropriate outlet for instinctual drives, particularly among the 'lower classes', and that this had led to a wide range of social problems including 'nervous strain'.

As well as providing a naturalized justification for social inequalities and behaviour, Darwinism also gave rise to the eugenics movement which merged evolutionary theory with an earlier Malthusian[15] agenda of population control. The eugenicists believed that modern society was undermining the natural selection process by protecting the weak and 'degenerate' (particularly among the poor), allowing them to reproduce more rapidly than the middle and upper classes. Marie Stopes, an early advocate of contraception for the poor, was motivated by this moral panic about 'racial degeneration'.[16] However, the eugenics movement was not confined to a narrow pressure group, but was widely endorsed by the European intelligentsia, even among those who considered themselves progressive, for example, the Bloomsbury group.[17]

Social Darwinism and the eugenics movement reached their zenith in the pre-war period when Cannon and Selye were laying the foundations of the stress discourse and they had a fundamental impact on the way in which the subject was approached, studied and theorized at this time.

Walter Cannon was Professor of Physiology at Harvard University and his interests lay in the physiological changes that occurred in response to environmental stimuli. Cannon was involved in a series of laboratory experiments at Harvard which were reported in various medical and physiology journals and summarized in his book, *Bodily Changes in Pain, Hunger, Fear and Rage*, published in 1925.[18] In the Darwinist tradition, Cannon felt that the 'emotions' listed in the title of his book were essentially biologically determined 'instincts' which had evolved over aeons of human adaptation to environmental threats. As such, these instincts were of adaptive value in the struggle for survival:

In the long history of the race . . . there have been savage creatures, human and subhuman, watching with stealth and ready to attack without a moment's warning. And there has also been the necessity of fighting, for revenge, for safety and for prey. In that harsh school fear and anger have served as a preparation for action. Fear has become associated with the instinct to run, to escape; and anger or aggressive feeling, with the instinct to attack. These are fundamental emotions and instincts which have resulted from the experience of multitudes of generations in the fierce struggle for existence and which have their values in that struggle.[19]

From this highly Darwinian point of departure Cannon developed his theory of the fight or flight response to explain the physiological changes that take place in the stressed[20] body. The outward manifestations of the fight or flight response (including pallor, cold sweat, dry mouth, rapid heartbeat and respiration and physical shaking) were already commonly recognized, but Cannon was interested in the physiological changes that occurred beneath the surface of the body and which could not, therefore, be easily observed. The response of the adrenal system proved fundamental, flooding the body with adrenaline when confronted by an environmental threat.

This rush of adrenaline was found to have a number of specific effects on the body including the release of stored carbohydrate from the liver to provide a burst of energy to the heart, lungs, brain and limbs and increasing the rate at which the blood coagulates. These changes prepared the body to fight or take flight (or to heal a physical injury rapidly in the case of blood coagulation). A more detailed account of the physiological changes that comprise the stress response is given below. Here we are concerned not so much with Cannon's empirical observations, but with the theoretical framework in which he interpreted them, and, more specifically, the extent to which that theoretical framework was a product of the prevailing intellectual climate and the influence that it has had on subsequent conceptions of stress in both scientific and popular discourses.

The principal component of Cannon's explanation of the fight or flight response was essentially a Darwinian model of evolutionary adaptation to environmental threats. Thus, the physiological changes that comprised the stress response were viewed as the result of evolutionary pressures, by which those who were best able to act decisively in response to an environmental threat (literally by fighting or taking flight) were more likely to survive and reproduce than those who lacked such adaptive characteristics. So for Cannon what came to be described as the stress response was not only positive, but an essential element of human survival. There is little indication in Cannon's writings that the stress response might have a harmful effect on physical or mental health. And it is here that Cannon is most at odds with contemporary stress discourse where the emphasis is very much on the adverse consequences of stress.

The closest Cannon came to suggesting that stress might have adverse physiological consequences was in his account of the economy of the stressed body, which he described in terms of a country preparing for war:

> Just as in war between nations the arts and industries which have brought wealth and contentment must suffer serious neglect or be wholly set aside both by the attacker and the attacked, and all the supplies and energies developed in the period of peace must be devoted to the pursuit of conflict; so, likewise, the functions which in quiet times establish and support the bodily reserves are, in times of stress, instantly checked or completely stopped, and these reserves lavishly drawn upon to increase power in the attack and in the defence or flight.[21]

In the aftermath of the First World War this metaphor must have seemed particularly apt, but Cannon did not explore the possibility that a diversion of bodily resources towards action and away from routine repair work might have pathological effects. One reason for this omission is Cannon's interest in the 'homeostasis' of the body, i.e. the processes by which the body maintains a relatively steady internal state under widely varying environmental conditions: for example, body temperature remains relatively constant regardless of changes in climate.

In his later work,[22] Cannon explored the processes that ensure homeostasis including the role of the parasympathetic nervous system in reversing the physiological changes that comprise the stress response and return the body to a steady state. Cannon's commitment to the principle of homeostasis left no room for the possibility that the stress response might be harmful. The physiological changes that comprise the fight or flight response were short-lived adaptive responses and, therefore, in Cannon's opinion unlikely to cause lasting harm.

Cannon's description of the stressed body shifting resources away from maintenance and repair towards immediate action remains a very dominant theme in contemporary endocrinological and immunological accounts of the stress response. However, the physiologists that came after Cannon were less sanguine about the body's capacity for maintaining homeostasis and (as discussed below) have compiled evidence of the health problems that can be caused by chronic stress.

For Cannon, the problem lay not so much in a surfeit of stressors, so much as the limited opportunities for exercising the 'fighting instinct' in modern society. After Graham Wallas[23] (whom he cites),[24] Cannon was concerned that failure to exercise the fighting spirit might lead to physical and moral degeneration. However, despite his belief in the morally uplifting experience of war, Cannon felt that modern warfare was simply too barbarous to tolerate and that the martial spirit should be cultivated either through competitive sport or against enemies such as 'pain, disease, poverty and sin'.[25]

Cannon's defence of the martial spirit (if not of actual war) is perhaps the most dated element of his work, reflecting a time when the militarist certainties of the nineteenth century were still in circulation, even if they were increasingly brought into question by the experience of modern warfare. Today military conflict is legitimated by a quite different ideology[26] which emphasizes 'peace keeping' and the enforcement of international law rather than the satisfaction of a 'fighting instinct'. Similarly, the critique of masculinity and growing emphasis on emotional expressivity have served to pathologize aggression (see Chapter 4). Even so, the broader theme of modern society at odds with 'nature', or at least with the biological legacy of evolution, remains a dominant theme within contemporary discourse; and the image of the modern individual whose 'stone age' instinctual drives and physiological responses are frustrated by, and inappropriate for, modern life remains a dominant perspective in many contemporary accounts of the stress phenomenon.

Despite Cannon's defence of the 'martial virtues' as an essential means of tackling challenges and problems faced at the individual and collective levels, he failed to recognize the role of personal resilience (or, indeed, of cognition generally) in mediating the fight or flight response. The relationship between environmental stressor and physiological response was felt to be automatic and the mediating role of social and psychological factors was largely ignored. The experience of fear or rage was simply another biological state akin to pain or hunger, occurring in response to the presence or absence of particular stimuli.[27] Although these reflexes were purposive (i.e. acting in the organism's interests by protecting against injury), they were activated automatically like other reflexes such as swallowing, vomiting or coughing. Thus, there is no suggestion in Cannon's work that the fight or flight response might be governed by the individual's assessment of the environmental threat or his or her capacity to tackle it.

As we saw in Chapter 1, the belief that stress is not mediated by consciousness remains a common theme in many contemporary representations of the work stress phenomenon, for instance in the trade unionists' claim that 'employers [who] damage the minds of their employees . . . will have to pay out in the same way as if they did not repair the stairs and someone fell down and broke a leg'.[28] However, other representations of work stress emphasize the role of 'personality' or 'psychological factors' in the mediation of work stress, and, as we shall see below, this has been the major theme of psychological research into stress.

Cannon's focus on the physiological changes that comprise the fight or flight response, and his failure to examine the processes that mediate the relationship between stressor and response, mean that his conception of stress is quite different to the psycho-social model that currently prevails. Similarly, his insistence that the fight or flight response is a wholly positive reflex contributing to the organism's health and welfare (rather than a cause of mental and physical illness) would at best only receive qualified support from most contemporary physiologists. These factors locate Cannon's work in the prehistory of stress, even though his conception of the fight or flight response still forms the basis of physiological accounts of the stress response.

The next step in the emergence of stress as a scientific construct can be found in the work of the endocrinologist Hans Selye. As a young medical student in 1920s Prague, and as an endocrinological researcher at McGill University, Montreal, in the 1930s, Selye was a product of the same cultural and intellectual climate that had shaped Cannon's approach. However, although the two physiologists shared a common point of departure, across the course of his career Selye developed a much broader conception of stress which included an account of its negative effects on health. Moreover, Selye was a tireless promoter of the stress concept, whose efforts, more than those of anyone else in the field, served to embed the notion firmly in the popular and scientific imagination.[29]

In his own accounts, Selye emphasized that he had 'discovered' stress almost by accident.[30] While conducting laboratory experiments on rats, in order to study female sex hormones, Selye found that whatever tissue extracts he administered into his rats, the same physiological responses occurred – atrophy of the thymus and lymphatic system and ulceration of intestines and the adrenal cortex. Selye concluded that his experiments must be contaminated and gave up in despair. However, as a result of this experience Selye began to postulate the theory of a non-specific physiological response to 'noxious agents' in the environment.[31]

Initially, Selye referred to the noxious agents as stress, but later used the term to describe the state of the organism in adaptation to the environment. Like Cannon before him, Selye couched his stress theory within a Darwinian framework which emphasized the struggle to adapt and survive in a hostile environment, and called his theory the General Adaptation Syndrome (GAS). The GAS involved a three-stage process of physiological adaptation: alarm – akin to Cannon's fight or flight response, in which the body reacts strongly to an external threat; resistance – in which the body's reactions appear to return to normal, but resources are still being taxed, leaving the body vulnerable to disease; and exhaustion – when the body's resources for combating stress have been all but used up and the continual stress is likely to have serious health consequences and may possibly lead to death. Selye described the health problems associated with the stress response as 'diseases of adaptation', and felt that he had discovered one of the fundamental mechanisms of health and illness.

The GAS is an expansion of Cannon's fight or flight response, predicting what will happen if an environmental stressor is not dealt with in the short term but continues to challenge the organism. Like Cannon, Selye believed that some forms of stress could be good for the organism (he described them as eustress), but his most significant contribution to the stress discourse was the association between stress and ill health, or the 'pathologization of stress'.[32] This marked a major transition from Cannon's earlier position and triggered an agenda that continues to dominate research and popular discourse.

A second discursive development that is usually attributed to Selye is the inclusion of psychological stressors into the field. Like Cannon, Selye's early experimental research had been solely concerned with physical stressors including heat, cold, forced exercise, electric shock, x-ray exposure, etc., all of which appeared to produce the same physiological changes. However, in his later work Selye broadened the list of potential stressors to include psychological and emotional stressors:

> The soldier who sustains wounds in battle, the mother who worries about her soldier son, the gambler who watches the races, the horse and the jockey he bet on; they are all under stress . . . The housewife who tries to keep her children out of trouble, the child who scalds himself . . . they too are under stress. This is a fundamental question in the life of everyone; it touches closely upon the essence of life and disease.[33]

This expansion of stress theory came about not just as a result of Selye's experimental work, but because of the role of the Second World War in promoting interest in psychological stressors. As well as providing additional empirical evidence to inform his theorizing, the war also enabled Selye to recruit the support of the military establishment in promoting stress research in the immediate post-war period.[34–5] As Viner[36] has observed, it was Selye's ability to forge alliances with the military (and other powerful groups) that played a key role in the promotion of stress theory, rather than the support of his colleagues in academic physiology who were for the most part critical of his work.

The military interest in stress psychology stemmed partly from concern about civilian and military morale and psycho-neuroses,[37-40] partly from the desire to develop offensive techniques,[41] but mainly in order to aid in the recruitment and training of combat personnel, particularly those who would be involved in covert operations behind enemy lines and who might, therefore, face interrogation or even torture.[42-4] As well as stimulating research, the military interest in stress also led to the development of a research infrastructure in the post-war period, including the Neuropsychiatric Division of the Walter Reed Army Medical Center in Washington, DC; the Military Stress Laboratory of the US Army; the Naval Medical Research Unit; the Stress and Hypertension Clinic of the Naval Gun Factory, and the Stress Medicine Division of the Naval Health Research Centre. By the mid-1970s over a third of stress researchers were based in US military institutions.[45]

Selye tapped into the growing military interest in research, securing a position as expert consultant in stress to the Surgeon General of the US Army from 1947–57, and developing his stress theory to accommodate psychological stressors. Indeed, in the post-war period it was with the community of psychologists, rather than his colleagues in endocrinology, that Selye developed the greatest affinity and in 1950 he was invited to address the American Psychological Association, triggering widespread, though largely uncritical, use of the term among the profession.[46]

Selye also promoted his stress theory among other constituencies, including glossy magazines such as *Time* and the *Reader's Digest*, physicians, alternative therapists, and key figures on the Republican right.[47] As with Cannon's pronouncements a generation earlier, Selye's interpretation of stress reflected the social and political climate of the time. However, rather than reflecting the eugenicist's concern with the 'degeneration of the race', Selye's approach addressed the ideological imperatives of the cold war:

> For the Republican luminaries that Selye recruited to the board of the American Institute of Stress, such as Senators Barry Goldwater and Samuel Hayakawa, and the popular comedian Bob Hope, stress theory justified the position of the worker in capitalist society, and provided a means to deflect revolutionary and destructive tendencies into useful, natural worker activity.[48]

According to Viner,[49] it was Selye's ability to provide practical and ideological support to the American military–industrial complex, coupled with his tireless efforts to promote stress theory to the public (*The Stress of Life* was translated into 14 languages), that eventually prompted the assimilation of the stress category into scientific discourse. Rather than a well-validated scientific discovery slowly permeating popular consciousness, it was support for the concept among the masses and their growing tendency to interpret their experiences in terms of 'stress' that led to its gradual acceptance by what had previously been a highly sceptical scientific community.

By the late 1960s, largely as a result of Selye's proselytizing and support from the military, stress research had become well established in a number of centres, particularly among the psychological disciplines. However, the rapid growth in stress research did not represent a homogeneous research programme based on shared assumptions and a common theoretical framework, but rather a diverse range of perspectives, often using the category imprecisely and inconsistently. While Selye had placed stress on the public and scientific agenda, he failed to establish an authoritative definition of the term, or impose a uniform theoretical hegemony, not least because his own empirical research and that of Cannon before him had been largely discredited by subsequent physiologists. Thus, by the close of the decade there were a number of competing stress theories, particularly within psychology. While a detailed survey of all the different strands of post-war stress research is not possible here, what follows is a summary of the key approaches that have shaped contemporary stress discourse.

A common thread in the scientific discourse of stress is the relationship between the individual and the environment. However, although most theorists have recognized the importance of both, they vary considerably in the amount of explanatory power they ascribe to each. Thus, in the post-war period there appears to be a bifurcation between those who focused mainly on the attributes of the individual, such as personality traits, and those who were mainly concerned with the situational or environmental 'causes' of stress. Again, these differences in emphasis represent changing cultural and political contexts.

A key aspect of the stress research that focused on individual characteristics (rather than environmental influences) was a concern with how stress might affect task performance. As noted above, this theme originated during the Second World War, with attempts by the military to recruit resilient staff and bolster their performance in battle. This concern continued in the post-war period; for instance the US air force funded a major programme of laboratory research into the effects of stress on task performance, led by Richard Lazarus.[50-1] The military's concern to optimize the task performance of its personnel under stressful conditions coincides with the industrialists' concern to maximize the productivity of workers,[52-3] and throughout the post-war period stress researchers have continued to respond to the demands of the military–industrial complex by developing a range of psychological tests and procedures which aim to bolster performance under stress through effective recruitment and training of staff.[54]

Research into stress and human performance provided an empirical and theoretical base for the burgeoning human resource management movement, giving rise to a particular focus on *work* stress rather than stress in general. Throughout the 1960s and 1970s the field was dominated by role stress theorists at the University of Michigan. The Michigan school can be traced back to 1947, but it was a study published in 1964[55] that really established role theory, prompting a huge programme of research that was still yielding academic publications in the late 1980s.[56] Role theory was heavily influenced by the social psychology of Kurt Lewin,[57] reflected in an emphasis on individual perceptions and expectations rather than the extent to which roles are determined by social structure and other external constraints.[58] One of the earlier role theory studies looked at the Prudential Insurance Company and found that the role of the supervisor was central to team performance, citing avoidance of over-supervision and an emphasis on the needs of the worker rather than just on production as key factors in the amelioration of stress.[59] Subsequent role theory studies largely maintained this focus on leadership, role conflict and organizational structure, neglecting broader social structural factors. The highly individualized conception of role stress effectively depoliticized the work stress discourse, facilitating its easy passage into corporate human resource management. Thus, role theory was both a product of the particular historical conjuncture in which it emerged, i.e. the military–industrial agenda of cold-war America, and a major contributor to the emerging work stress discourse.

While the role theorists were building their hegemonic dominance of the work stress discourse in North America, across the Atlantic a radically different approach to the phenomenon was emerging. The Scandinavian approach to work stress developed in a quite different political context to that of its North American counterpart, reflecting a Social Democratic agenda of work reform and industrial democracy that was supported by the trade union movement as well as by government and employers' organizations. This progressive political climate gave rise to a quite different research focus which concentrated on work characteristics and occupational health, rather than on the subjective experiences of the worker and task performance. The primary aim was to improve working conditions and morale, rather than simply boost productivity.

A key figure in Scandinavian stress research is Bertil Gardell who suggested that jobs which entailed relatively little worker autonomy or skill use tended to be associated with poor mental health.[60] This focus on work characteristics and their effect on mental health and well-being developed through the 1970s and 1980s; for instance, the Swedish National Board of Occupational Safety and Health funded a study of working conditions in the sawmill industry, which found that workers who reported job monotony, high attention demands and psychological strain were more likely to suffer psychosomatic illness and absenteeism than a control group.[61–2] This epidemiological approach to exploring the relationship between work characteristics and mental and physical health was taken up by a broad range of researchers both in Europe and the United States, most notably in the work of Robert Karasek and Thores Theorell,[63] a more detailed account of which is given below. However, although the lineage of many contemporary epidemiological accounts of work stress can be traced back to Gardell and the Scandinavian work reform movement the political content of the approach has changed significantly, from an emphasis on the social democratic agenda of industrial democracy towards a more individualized focus on human resource management, health promotion and litigation.

This transformation is partly attributable to a broader historical decline in trade union militancy and the post-war social democratic ideology of western governments, but can also be viewed as a consequence of the way in which the relationship between work characteristics and health was conceptualized by researchers adopting an epidemiological approach. Thus, at the height of the work reform movement in the 1960s and 1970s the findings of researchers such as Gardell had a direct impact upon legislation which was designed to change the balance of power between employer and employee, such as the Norwegian Work Environment Act and the Swedish Act of Co-determination. These measures appear to have been of limited effectiveness,[64] suggesting that the conflict of interests between labour and capital cannot be easily resolved by legal administrative measures. This, coupled with the rise of neo-liberalism and the demise of trade union militancy, effectively closed the Scandinavian approach to work reform.[65] However, the epidemiological approach that informed the work reform movement remains influential even though it has been largely shorn of its social democratic content.

As the analysis presented in Chapter 1 illustrates, the assumption of a direct relationship between work characteristics (such as low levels of job control or social support) and poor physical or mental health, without reference to consciousness or other mediating factors, remains a common theme in trade union and government contributions to the work stress discourse. The difference is that work stress has been transformed from a political issue into an occupational health concern. Rather than pointing towards the need for a radical restructuring of production relations the epidemiology of work stress now implies the need for employers to protect the health of their workers by adopting effective strategies of human resource management and providing appropriate therapy or compensation where such measures fail. This depoliticization of work stress stems not just from the broader decline of radical and social democratic politics, but from the way in which the phenomenon has been conceived by epidemiologists. Rather than conceiving of the worker as an active social agent in a specific political and historical context, epidemiologists have constructed the 'work stress victim' as a subject within medical discourse, i.e. as someone suffering a disease. In this sense the worker is no longer a political agent struggling for better working conditions as an end in themselves, but a vulnerable 'body' to be protected from hazards in the working environment which might cause physical or mental illness. The political struggle to overcome powerlessness and alienation is transformed into a health and safety issue in which 'job demands', 'decision latitude', 'skill discretion' and 'social support' have a purely aetiological significance.

It is not simply the case that the epidemiological conception of work stress constitutes a mystification of political issues, or the pursuit of political objectives by other means – the end point is not political emancipation but a healthy and, therefore, more productive workforce.

In the first half of this chapter we have presented a brief history of the emergence of work stress as a scientific category, charting the key perspectives that have shaped this discourse. Although the different approaches have been presented in roughly chronological order, it would be wrong to assume that this represents a linear course of development in which evidence has gradually accrued and theoretical insights have been progressively refined or rejected. In fact the scientific discourse of work stress remains extremely diverse, with a wide range of competing perspectives. As late as 1981 the United States National Research Council inquiry into stress research found different and conflicting definitions of the phenomenon, a lack of scientific rigour and conceptual confusion.[66]

The historical analysis presented above illustrates the extent to which the scientific discourse of work stress has developed in response to changing political, ideological and cultural concerns. From the neo-Darwinism of Cannon and Selye, through the military and industrial concerns of the cold war with their emphasis on human performance, up to the social democratic and post-social democratic agenda of the Scandinavian epidemiologists, stress has provided a sufficiently amorphous, yet consistently meaningful, category through which these concerns could be addressed. Yet it would be wrong to conclude that stress is therefore pure invention. The very fact that the category has such a powerful and persistent hold on both the public and scientific imagination suggests that it must at least partially grasp the reality of lived experience. While we would reject the 'Whig history' of stress which suggests that the phenomenon has an objective 'truth' which was 'discovered' by rigorous scientific inquiry, we would also question the strong social constructionist argument which suggests that epistemological considerations are irrelevant, for example, Foucault's claim that

> the problem does not consist in drawing the line between that in a discourse which falls under the category of scientificity or truth, and that which comes under some other category, but in seeing historically how effects of truth are produced within discourses which in themselves are neither true nor false.[67]

As the history of medical knowledge indicates, establishing the truth or falsity of a proposition is essential to the pursuit of health, happiness and well-being.[68] While scientific inquiry may not offer a means of arriving at absolute truths, it does at least offer a means of evaluating the extent to which truth claims are supported by empirical evidence, even if this process is often distorted by poor methodology, overly speculative theorizing, and by the influence of vested interests.[69] In this sense, it is not sufficient simply to illustrate the extent to which a discourse like work stress is influenced by the social, cultural and political context in which it was produced, or the extent to which this body of knowledge influenced the ways in which people subsequently interpreted and gave meaning to their experiences. Historical deconstruction of this kind must be dovetailed with a more formal appraisal of the epistemological status of the discourse, even though it is recognized that analysis of this kind cannot arrive at absolute truths, but only an assessment of what appears to be most likely given the available evidence. To this end the analysis now turns to an appraisal of the current 'state of the art' research and theory in work stress. The evidence will be presented under three broad themes to which several disciplines and sub-disciplines have contributed: epidemiology, physiology and psychology.

The epidemiology of work stress

It is the epidemiological approach to work stress which has had the most fundamental impact upon the public discourse described in Chapter 1. Both start from the assumption that, if not actually a disease in itself, work stress is a major cause of illness, and that the problem is sufficiently widespread to constitute an epidemic. The disease paradigm of work stress which exercises such a powerful grip on both the public and epidemiological imagination implies that the phenomenon operates largely independently of the conscious thoughts of the individual or the social and cultural factors that shape them. Thus, the pathway from adverse circumstances, through physiological and psychological distress, to illness, is often presented as an autonomous process which mirrors the germ theory of infectious disease, i.e. as a direct consequence of exposure to particular environmental conditions. From this perspective, adverse experiences at work are treated as objectively pathogenic agents, capable of generating disease regardless of the interpretation put upon them by the individual – stressors simply invade the body and cause disease.

Despite the large number of epidemiological studies of work stress and their potent influence on public perceptions of the phenomenon, it is a standpoint which is becoming increasingly difficult to sustain in the face of mounting theoretical criticisms and contradictory empirical evidence. Rather than abandon the epidemiological approach, attempts have been made to broaden its scope to include some aspects of the individual's interpretations, meanings and beliefs. However, it will be argued that rather than bolstering the epidemiological approach these additions and modifications are points on a trajectory which inevitably leads away from the epidemiological approach.

One of the first requirements of the epidemiological approach to work stress is to find out how many people are affected by it. A valid and reliable prevalence rate has proven elusive however, with different studies yielding substantially different estimates of the problem.[70-1] In response to the uncertainty regarding prevalence rates for work stress the Health and Safety Executive commissioned what was hoped to be a definitive study of the problem. The Bristol Stress and Health at Work Study[72] aimed to 'determine the prevalence and severity of occupational stress in a random population sample', and to 'distinguish stress caused by work from that caused by other factors'. In order to address the methodological difficulties of earlier studies self-reported data on work stress were 'validated' by the use of biochemical assays, measures of health-related behaviour, and by controlling for 'negative affect'. As a further check, the study adopted a two-stage design, repeating the measurements after twelve months.

The main measurement of work stress was achieved by asking respondents (n = 7069) to a postal survey to indicate whether they found their job: not at all stressful, mildly stressful, moderately stressful, very stressful or extremely stressful. The findings were broadly the same for the initial survey and the twelve-month follow-up, with 15–16 per cent describing their job as stressful and 2–3 per cent as extremely stressful, giving a combined prevalence rate of 18 per cent. Respondents in the high-stress group were more likely to report adverse work characteristics such as high demands, long hours, shiftwork, or exposure to physical stressors such as noise, and to report health-related behaviours such as little exercise, more frequent alcohol consumption, tobacco smoking and poor diet. 'Stressed' workers were also more likely to report higher rates of chronic ill health, general practitioner consultations, and sick leave. A small cohort study (n = 188) used more detailed measures (e.g. the Occupational Stress Indicator) to validate the subjective reports of stress. The personality trait of negative affectivity was also measured and many of the associations between stress and health remained after controlling for this variable and for high general life stress. Physiological tests (including blood test and salivary cortisol) were also conducted but did not yield clinically significant variations between high- and low-stress groups.

The findings of the Bristol study appear to confirm many of the key themes of the work stress discourse: that a substantial proportion of the workforce is affected by it, and that it has consequences for health-related behaviour as well as for physical and psychological health. A number of grey areas in the work stress debate also appear to be clarified; for instance, it is suggested that the effects of work stress can be distinguished from those of other stressors, and that the relationship between self-reported work characteristics and health is not simply a product of gloomy people making an unreasonably negative assessment of both. But are these appearances and conclusions valid? Despite the size of the sample used and its multifaceted research design the Bristol study can be criticized on a number of points.

Most obviously, the response rate of 49 per cent raises the question of how representative the findings are of the broader population; a particularly pertinent question given the intention of establishing a robust prevalence rate. In their defence, the authors demonstrate that the group of respondents shared many of the socio-demographic characteristics of the population from which they were drawn, but this is far from a guarantee that their experiences of work stress were representative. Those for whom work stress was not a problem may have found the questionnaire irrelevant and, therefore, been less likely to return it (leading to an inflated prevalence rate among respondents), or those experiencing severe job strain may have been too busy to complete the questionnaire (leading to an underestimate of prevalence). Another issue which may have inflated the prevalence rate is the extent to which respondents were 'primed' by the title of the questionnaire. McManus et al.,[73] in their study of the medical profession, found that the prevalence rate for work stress was substantially inflated when respondents were made aware that the study was about stress, perhaps reflecting a tendency for respondents to provide researchers with the evidence that they think they are looking for – the title of the 'Bristol Stress and Health Study' appeared twice on the cover of the questionnaire and at the head of each page therein.

The problem of arriving at a reliable prevalence rate is compounded by a more significant concern about what is actually being measured. If respondents are asked to state how many cigarettes they usually smoke in a week, the chances are that they will at least understand what they are being asked (even if they are unwilling or unable to give an accurate answer); but such an assumption cannot be made when asking about stress. As we have seen, the stress category is extremely vague and amorphous within both the scientific and lay discourses. In Chapters 1 and 3 we report findings from our own research which has shown a wide range of definitions in use by workers. For some stress referred to how stimulating or challenging their job was, for example, 'It is what makes me get out of bed in the morning'; for others stress referred to unpleasant, but not particularly significant, aspects of their work, while for others it was seen as a major problem which posed a threat to their health and well-being. As with scientific accounts of work stress there were quite different interpretations of whether work stress was about the objective characteristics of the job, the attributes of the individual or the relationship between the two. The high degree of heterogeneity found in lay (and scientific) definitions of the work stress phenomenon suggests that a simple question like 'how stressful do you find your job?' cannot be relied upon to yield findings which are valid, i.e. to measure what it is intended to measure. This is partly because the question draws no distinction between the intensity and duration of stress – many jobs may make fairly constant demands upon the worker, but others vary a great deal; for instance, work in a hospital accident and emergency department may entail relatively rare episodes of extreme demands, interspersed by hours of thumb-twiddling boredom: does this make it a stressful job?

Not only did the Bristol study rely on such a question, it asked respondents to calibrate their answers by stating whether they found their job to be 'not at all', 'mildly', 'moderately', 'very', or 'extremely' stressful. We might concede that there is a significant difference between the extremes of the continuum, but it is surely a mistake to assume that the distinction between 'mildly stressful' and 'moderately stressful' or between 'very stressful' and 'extremely stressful' can consistently pick up genuine differences in the experiences reported, particularly given the lack of clarity about what is actually being measured. Despite these concerns the Bristol study used the question to assign respondents to high-stress and low-stress groups as a basis for statistically analysing the relationship between work stress and health.

The high- and low-stress groups identified using the above question were cross-tabulated with a number of other variables felt to be indicative of work stress, including job demands, chronic illness, and health-related behaviours, all of which were found to be significant. But do these associations really mean that poor health and unhealthy behaviour are caused by adverse work characteristics as the work stress thesis suggests? There are several reasons why this conclusion cannot safely be drawn. First, it may be that negative assessments of work characteristics and work stress are the result (rather than the cause) of poor mental and/or physical health, i.e. either by a direct influence on the type of work experiences to which individuals are exposed, or by making work more difficult to cope with.

Closely related to this problem is the role played by negative affectivity. The concept of negative affectivity is derived from psychological accounts of personality, but the concept is also pertinent to epidemiological studies of work stress because it has been suggested that it may confound the apparent relationships between job stressors and strains. Negative affectivity (NA) has been defined as a generalized tendency to view the world and oneself in negative terms.[74–5] Rather than a passing mood or reaction to particular circumstances NA (often also referred to as neuroticism) is allegedly one of the 'big five' personality dimensions, and is therefore felt to be a disposition which is relatively constant over time.[76] Those with high NA are more likely to experience distress and dissatisfaction, dwell more on their shortcomings, and be more dissatisfied with the world and with themselves than are individuals with low NA. Thus it is argued that high NA would predispose respondents to self-report higher levels of work-related stressors and higher rates of job strains, i.e. negative affective states, and that associations between self-reported stressors and strains would, therefore, be inflated.[77–9]

There are a number of conceptual issues around the characterization of NA as a stable disposition or personality dimension, not least of which is how it develops over time, and the problem (both conceptual and methodological) of distinguishing between NA as a long-term personality trait and relatively short-term emotional state triggered by particular circumstances (the trait–state dilemma). It has been suggested that NA may have a genetic component,[80] but this does not fully explain how NA develops over the life course in response to social experiences. If we accept the argument that NA is a stable personality trait, this raises the question of when this trait becomes 'fixed': is it predetermined before birth and therefore unaffected by positive and negative experiences, is it shaped by childhood experiences, becoming fixed during the transition to adulthood, or can prolonged and intense exposure to either positive or negative experiences modify trait NA at any point in the life course? This is a particularly vexing dilemma for those studying work stress, because many of the characteristics of NA (anxiety, depression, low self-esteem, etc.) are claimed to be indicators of job strain, making it difficult to distinguish between the output variable of psychological symptoms and the potentially confounding role played by NA.

Many studies have attempted to resolve this dilemma by drawing a sharp distinction between trait NA (the confounder) and state NA (the output variable). Trait NA is defined as that which is stable over a long period of time, and state NA as relatively short-term mental distress which may be caused by work. Trait NA can then be measured independently and the extent of its role as a confounding variable in the relationship between job stressors and strains can be determined through ever more complicated statistical analyses.[81–2] This was the approach taken in the cohort stage of the Bristol Stress and Health at Work Study, in which the Spielberger Trait Anxiety Inventory (STAI)[83] was used to measure NA. While some effects were no longer significant many of the associations between stress and health remained after controlling for the potentially confounding influence of NA.[84]

Although the statistical evidence from the Bristol study suggests that the confounding role of NA is modest, the assumptions on which this analysis is based can be questioned. First, the trait inventory of the STAI contains several components from the state inventory, for example 'I feel pleasant' and 'I feel rested', the only difference being that the state inventory asks about the intensity of these feelings at a given point in time, whereas the trait inventory asks about their frequency. Other items on the trait inventory refer to feelings which might more readily be recognized as long-term personality characteristics, e.g. 'I lack self-confidence', but even here it could be argued that someone experiencing a high degree of state NA (in response to a particular experience in or outside work) would be more likely to exaggerate their responses on the trait inventory, i.e. someone experiencing a brief state of anxiety may overestimate the extent to which they are generally prone to anxiety. And even if it is possible to distinguish a relatively long-term trait of NA from short-term NA states, can it be assumed that this 'personality dimension' is immune to social experiences across the life course (particularly experiences at work, given the amount of time spent at work and its important role in determining financial and emotional rewards)?

Thus, at a conceptual level it is extremely difficult to compartmentalize negative feelings into two mutually exclusive categories, the first of which represents a fixed personality trait that is largely independent of experiences at work and the second of which is a short-term state which may be caused by experiences at work. How long can a state of NA last before it is transformed into a trait? The STAI resolves this question by distinguishing between 'how you feel right now' and 'how you generally feel', but even long-term negative feelings must also exist at specific points in time, and emotional states which last for several months might be interpreted by respondents as how they feel 'generally', even though such states hardly constitute a personality dimension. And why is it that a cause (such as work stress) can be attributed to states of NA, but that the NA trait is considered to be independent of such causes? If a distinction cannot be drawn between NA as a state and a trait (and we would argue such a distinction cannot logically be made) then it would clearly be a mistake to claim that NA is autonomous, i.e. that it is not influenced by ongoing social experiences. This in turn necessarily leads to a more complex formulation of the relationship between NA and work stress. Rather than conceptualizing NA as either an effect of work stress or as a confounding variable in the relationship between stressors and strains, it is important to recognize the constantly interactive relationship between experiences at work and negative feelings – negative feelings may be caused by work stress (or any other social experience) but these negative feelings may themselves lead to an overly pessimistic assessment of both work characteristics and their effects on the individual. Studies which aim to 'control for' the confounding effects of NA by conjuring up a false trait–state dichotomy to which complicated statistical techniques can be applied represent an attempt to reduce the complexity of interactions between social experience and emotional life to the narrow constraints of the linear cause and effect relationship.

The above methodological and conceptual concerns raise fundamental questions about whether or not it is possible to use self-report data to obtain a prevalence rate for work stress. Asking people how stressful they find their jobs does not yield evidence of the prevalence of psychological or physical disease, nor does it reveal the extent of exposure to a clearly defined and quantifiable pathogenic agent. What it does provide is a rather ambiguous survey of attitudes towards work. While this may be of sociological and political interest (particularly in time series), it says very little about the causation or spread of disease.

Other epidemiologists have circumvented the difficulties of establishing a prevalence rate for the amorphous category of work stress, by focusing instead on the relationship between particular work characteristics and patterns of psychological and physical illness. There are several models, but the analysis will concentrate on the two which have been most widely tested and which have had the greatest impact upon the public discourse. The first is Robert Karasek and Thores Theorell's Demands–Control–Support model (DCS),[85] which developed from Gardell's work described above and focuses exclusively on work characteristics. The second, developed by the German sociologist Johannes Siegrist, is called the Effort–Reward Imbalance model (ERI),[86] which attempts to supplement assessment of work characteristics with measures of the respondent's appraisal of reciprocity in the relationship between the effort put into work and the rewards it confers. It will be argued that although Siegrist's model is methodologically similar to that of Karasek and Theorell's (both have claimed that they are complementary), the inclusion of conscious appraisal in the pathway from job characteristics to distress and illness marks a fundamental break with the epidemiological standpoint and the assumptions on which it is based.

The DCS model proposes that job strain is likely to occur when a worker faces high job demands in combination with low social support from colleagues/managers and/or low job control. The job control variable comprises two components: decision authority (being able to choose when and how tasks are completed) and skill discretion (whether a job is boring or repetitive, and the extent to which skills can be used and developed).

The composition of the DCS model reflects the transformation of the production process during the first half of the twentieth century, when Henry Ford's popularization of the production line, coupled with Taylor's time and motion studies, transformed manufacturing industry. Rather than a skilled artisan with a relatively high degree of skill and autonomy, the factory worker became increasingly deskilled and subordinated to managerial control;[87] little more than a 'cog' in the production machine, as Chaplin graphically portrayed in his film *Modern Times*. Karasek and Theorell's model attempts to measure the extent of this dehumanizing shift in the organization of production to provide quantitative data which can be correlated with indicators of psychological well-being and physical health. The aim is to show that 'modern' production techniques are not only unpleasant for the worker but also a major cause of morbidity and premature mortality.

The DCS model has developed and expanded since it was first conceptualized in the early 1970s (for instance, the social support variable is a relatively recent addition).[88] However, the methodology behind it remains essentially the same. Workers are presented with a series of questions (about 27 depending on the version) all of which relate to either job demands, job control, or social support; for example, one of the questions relating to job control asks: 'Do you have to do the same thing over and over again?' Respondents are asked to tick one of four boxes to indicate whether they encounter a particular work characteristic 'often, sometimes, seldom, or, never'. The options are scored from 0 to 3 and all of the responses relating to a particular variable can then be aggregated giving individual scores for the three dimensions of the model.

The model has been tested many times, in different industries, occupational groups and geographical locations particularly in Scandinavia and the USA.[89–90] Many of the studies have measured the association between job strain and various indicators of anxiety and depression, for example, the General Health Questionnaire[91] is often used to yield quantitative data on psychiatric distress.[92] Other studies have looked at the relationship between job strain and physical diseases, particularly cardiovascular disease,[93] and behavioural variables such as sickness absence from work.[94] Not all of the studies confirm the predictions of the model,[95] and the tendency not to publish negative findings must always be borne in mind; even so there is sufficient evidence to suggest that an association between the DCS model of job strain and the above health and behavioural indicators can be supported – generally it seems that the greater the degree of job strain, the more likely an individual is to experience mental distress, depression, and a range of health problems, particularly cardiovascular disease. However, not all of the components of the DCS model are equally strong predictors of health outcomes; for example, in their review Schnall *et al.* found that 17 out of 25 studies reported a significant association between job control and cardiovascular outcomes, whereas the job demands variable was only a significant predictor in 8 out of 23.[96] That job control is the key component of the DCS, at least in predicting cardiovascular problems, has also been found in other studies,[97–8] including the British Whitehall II study.[99]

The Whitehall II study[100] of a cohort of over 10,000 male and female civil servants is one of the more rigorous attempts to test the relationship between the DCS model variables and health outcomes. The study combined self-report questionnaire data and independent assessments of work characteristics with a range of physiological tests. A longitudinal design was adopted and there have been five waves of data collection since the study commenced in 1985. Analysis of the first three waves of data yielded the following findings about the relationship between the DCS variables and health-related behaviour/health outcomes. All three variables were associated with poor mental health and poor health functioning. Low social support at work and low decision latitude were also related to increased sickness absence, and low decision latitude was also found to be associated with alcohol dependence. It was also found that the influence of work-related factors on health was as great as the influence of non-work-related factors.

The relationship between the DCS variables and coronary heart disease was also explored in the Whitehall II study.[101] It was found that although men and women with low job control had a higher risk (OR 1.5) of newly reported CHD over a mean five-year follow-up, job demands and social support at work were not related to the risk of new CHD. However, this may be attributable to the particular characteristics of the Whitehall workforce. Evidence from the SHEEP case control study in Stockholm suggests that high job demands combined with low control increase the risk of myocardial infarction in men.[102]

Thus, studies using Karasek and Theorell's DCS model of job strain have proved a rich source of evidence to inform perceptions of the relationship between work stress and illness, but is this evidence valid? It is certainly questionable on a number of counts. In many of the studies which have tested the model the measurement of work characteristics, and in some instances the measurements of health status as well, depend upon self-reported assessments made by the worker. This raises a number of problems, not least of which is the extent to which these reports may be influenced by factors independent of the workplace which may affect the individual's state of mind leading to an overly pessimistic assessment of both work characteristics and health. Thus, as with the Bristol study's attempt to use self-report data to find a prevalence rate for work stress, rather than adverse work characteristics causing psychological distress or illness, the causal relationship may run in the opposite direction, with a negative assessment of work characteristics resulting from 'negative affect', which in turn may result from illness or other factors which have little connection with the workplace.

There are essentially two approaches which attempt to overcome the difficulties associated with the use of self-report data. The first uses existing knowledge about the work characteristics associated with particular jobs to impute job characteristics to workers on the basis of their job titles.[103] This technique is particularly valuable in analysing large existing data sets which contain information on job title and health variables, but lack detailed data on job characteristics. More importantly, because the data on work characteristics are obtained from a different sample to that which is being studied there is arguably less of a problem with self-report bias or reverse causation. However, the technique is dependent upon accurate data on work characteristics obtained from other studies, sometimes by expert observer assessment of job characteristics (see below for criticism of this technique), or by the self-report technique. These data are used to find the mean levels of work characteristics associated with particular occupations. Averaging the individual scores reduces the influence of individual biases, but it does not overcome the problem of selection, i.e. the tendency for people with particular personality traits and life experiences to be recruited into particular occupations. Moreover the technique does not allow for variations in work characteristics between people with the same job title; for example, someone teaching in a deprived inner city comprehensive school may have substantially different experiences at work from those of a colleague at an affluent suburban school even though they have the same job title. Thus there is no guarantee that attributed work characteristics will accurately reflect the experiences of those to whom they are ascribed.

The second approach attempts to overcome self-report bias by using expert observers to assess job characteristics independently.[104] Superficially, this approach appears to offer an ideal solution to the problems associated with self-report data – they should (in theory) not be confounded by the personality of the worker and they can also take into account the specific organizational context of a job. However, the claimed 'objectivity' of such assessments can be questioned. First, who makes the assessment: is it a colleague/co-worker or a truly independent observer? In the former instance, the co-worker may be influenced as much by their colleague's behaviour and interpretation as they are by the objective work characteristics, while in the latter case the observer may not have sufficient exposure to each occupation to make an accurate appraisal of the work characteristics. Secondly, on what basis is the assessment made – archival data, work site observation, or an observational interview with the worker? Archival sources, such as the traffic density encountered by bus drivers, may be objective, but do they adequately grasp the full range of work characteristics associated with a particular occupation (and as they are usually collected for purposes other than research there is no guarantee of their accuracy)? Work site observations and interviews again run the risk of the observer's judgement being influenced by the behaviour and attitudes of the worker which may be due to factors outside work.

These attempts to overcome the constraints of self-report data are seductive, promising to provide an 'objective' basis for the study of the relationship between work characteristics and health, rather than relying on the subjective testimony of the worker. Surely, on average, the adverse work characteristics encountered by, say, a city centre bus driver will be greater than those encountered by a librarian or gardener, and surely these differences will be apparent to a trained observer? The problems begin when we move away from the extremes of the work stress continuum to the 'middle ground' where most occupations are found. Is general practice more stressful than hospital nursing? Is schoolteaching more demanding than social work? Do accountants have greater control over their work than estate agents? The claim that such differences can be objectively quantified is based on the epidemiological fallacy that pathogenic agents can be absolutely separated from the characteristics of the host. This may be valid in the case of an infectious disease like cholera or meningitis. It may even be appropriate to studies of physical or mental fatigue. But it becomes highly questionable when applied to the measurement of psycho-social stress, where the characteristics of the job and those of the individual worker are far more closely bound. Is it legitimate, on the basis of an 'objective' appraisal of work characteristics, to label a job as highly stressful, even though its incumbent exhibits no physical, psychological or behavioural symptoms and claims to be highly satisfied and happy with his or her work? And by the same token, if someone takes early retirement due to mental health problems putatively caused by work, even though colleagues doing 'objectively' the same job report no symptoms, should this be logged as another case of work stress? The point is that work stress (or job strain) does not reside exclusively in the objective characteristics of work, nor in the personal attributes of the individual, but in the relationship between the two – a relationship that is mediated by subjective interpretations and appraisal. Pursuit of the elusive objective measure of job strain is bound to fail because characteristics which one worker will find to be an unbearable burden will be experienced as a stimulating challenge by another.

In the Whitehall II study, self-report data on work characteristics were complemented with supposedly objective assessments conducted by personnel officers. The associations between job strain and ill health evaporated when the self-report data were replaced with the supposedly objective assessments, leading the researchers to conclude that: '. . . objective measures do not take into account the individual experience of being in the job and may have been relatively crude measures of control and demands at work'.[105] Other studies have had greater success in demonstrating an association between supposedly objective measures of job strain and health outcomes,[106] yet the methodological and conceptual issues raised above suggest that such 'objective' techniques are as questionable as the self-report techniques they were designed to underpin.

Even if the self-report and 'objective' measurements of work characteristics are an accurate reflection of the conditions that prevail in the workplace, they and the psychological and health problems they are associated with may be the product of social deprivation, i.e. those who are born into poverty may be more likely to end up in low-control/high-demands jobs, and their experiences of material deprivation may also lead to poor mental and physical health. In response to this criticism much has been made of the Whitehall study of civil servants which found that mortality rates in the most junior grades were three times higher than those in the most senior grades.[107] As Richard Wilkinson has suggested, the Whitehall study excluded the most deprived socio-economic classes and focused on white-collar workers who would probably define themselves as middle class.[108] Although there were substantial variations in income between the top and bottom grades, even the most junior staff were unlikely to be experiencing a degree of material deprivation that was likely to explain their relatively poor health status, thus it is argued that the role of material deprivation as a confounding variable in the relationship between work characteristics and health status can be discounted. However, as George Davey Smith[109] has suggested, this defence makes the mistake of assuming that the effects of deprivation on health are contemporaneous, when in fact deprivation in childhood may have health consequences which emerge throughout the life course.

Hence, although the junior civil servants in the Whitehall study may have escaped material deprivation through short-range social mobility, they may have been exposed to significant material deprivation in childhood, which in turn may have had consequences for their future health. That the junior grades were more likely to have encountered deprivation in childhood is demonstrated by the finding that their mean height was lower than that of the senior staff. To test for this potential effect the Whitehall researchers included height (as an indicator of childhood deprivation) in the regression models linking risk factors to CHD outcomes. While height (along with other risk factors) was found to have an effect, job control was still found to have an independent effect.[110] However, Davey Smith et al. have suggested that height is only a partial indicator of the socio-economic risk factors that deprived children are likely to encounter. When other factors are taken into consideration their effect on CHD outcomes is much greater and may account for the residual variations that have previously been attributed to job control and other psychological factors.[111–112] As with the Whitehall study, the substantial number of other studies which have found evidence of a relationship between job control and cardiovascular (and other) disease have not explored the effects of the full range of life course variables identified by Davey Smith et al., and it therefore remains to be seen whether this challenge to the apparent relationship between job control and health will be substantiated empirically.

Despite the substantial body of empirical evidence supporting the relationship between the DCS model variables and health outcomes there remain a number of methodological difficulties which have not been fully resolved: the reliance on self-report data; the potentially confounding role played by negative affectivity; the elusiveness of objective independent assessments of work characteristics; and the confounding role played by exposure to material deprivation across the life course. By themselves, these problems are sufficient to bring into question the apparent relationship between the DCS variables and health outcomes. However, there is also a fundamental conceptual issue that severely limits the explanatory range of Karasek and Theorell's approach.

The problem with the epidemiological concept of work stress is not just that the relationship between work characteristics and health outcomes is questionable on methodological grounds, but that it fails to grasp the role of consciousness in mediating that relationship. Karasek and Theorell's approach has been described as a 'black box' model of work stress[113] because it aims to demonstrate a statistical relationship between work characteristics and health outcomes without exploring the pathways between the input and output variables. Thus, while it might explain why certain working environments are particularly stressful, it does not account for why some people have the ability to withstand job strain (i.e. are resilient), while others do not and manifest psychological and somatic problems. The assumption is that high job demands, low job control and low social support are inherently pathogenic in the same way that, say, tobacco smoke is carcinogenic, i.e. at a purely biological level. It may well be that, for instance, a heavy workload causes physical fatigue, which may have direct and largely unconscious effects on the body; however, the job strain variables are not primarily concerned with fatigue, but with psychological stress, anxiety and depression. These experiences may be embodied (i.e. presenting themselves as physical symptoms, such as palpitations, headaches, sleeplessness etc.) and, therefore, measurable as physiological changes, but crucially they must also comprise an element of perception, cognition and reflection. Adverse experiences at work may provoke the 'fight or flight response' (see below), but in order for them to do so one must first perceive them as a threat. In Chapter 3 we look at the ways in which this relationship between an external stimulus and a physiological response can become embedded in the body over the life course and come to operate autonomously; however, the relationship must still be consciously learned in the first place. Moreover, once the stress mechanism has been triggered the individual must decide how to respond: fundamentally whether to fight, flee, or simply endure.

That the response to adverse experiences at work might entail both a subjective and social dimension has been partially recognized by Siegrist,[114] whose Effort–Reward Imbalance (ERI) model attempts to extend the epidemiological approach to work stress by incorporating some of the subjective assessments and interpretations made by the worker. The ERI model builds on the notion of job demands to include the amount of effort invested by the worker and suggests that mental distress and its health correlates arise when a high degree of effort is not reciprocated with adequate rewards in the form of pay, status and opportunities for advancement. A distinction is drawn between extrinsic effort (situational factors which make work more demanding) and intrinsic effort (personal factors such as motivation), and it is claimed a combination of both sources provides a more sensitive indicator of stress than Karasek and Theorell's model which only considers characteristics of the job. As with the DCS model the ERI model uses a list of questions with Likert scale response options (usually administered in a self-completion questionnaire) which can be scored and aggregated into variables.

As with the DCS model there is empirical evidence to support the ERI models; for instance, in the Whitehall II study effort–reward imbalance was found to be associated with increased risk of alcohol dependence, mental distress, sickness absence and poor health.[115] That empirical support can be found for both models raises a conceptual problem. Both approaches claim to explain job strain, yet, despite a common concern with the demands faced by the worker, the models also contain mutually exclusive variables; for instance, job control (supposedly the primary component of the DCS model) is not addressed in the ERI model. So how can both approaches fully explain the same phenomenon (job strain) when they comprise measures of different work characteristics?

One suggestion is that the two models may have distinctive contributions for explaining work stress for different types of occupation; for example,

Marmot *et al.*[116] suggest that effort–reward imbalance is frequent among service occupations and professions, in particular the ones dealing with person-based interactions (such as health professionals). Taken to its logical conclusion this argument leads to the inclusion of elements which are specific to particular jobs, i.e. the development of situation-specific models.[117] However, this introduces an element of arbitrariness regarding the organizational level at which work characteristics should be modelled; should they address particular industries, departments, occupations, or individual workers? The transition from a broadly generalizable model of job strain to one which is job- or worker-specific marks a move away from epidemiology towards biographical medicine. In effect this would amount to a deconstruction of the work stress phenomenon, raising the question of why stressors outside the workplace should not be included in such models.

Alternatively, it has been suggested that the models might be combined in order to enhance their explanatory power.[118] Evidence from a recent study of general practice confirmed that a combined model may perform better than either of the individual models, although there was no evidence to support the assumption that the ERI might be more powerful in service occupations.[119]

The strength of Siegrist's approach is that it begins to explore the subjective dimension of how work characteristics are interpreted by the worker. However, this innovation leaves the ERI model even more vulnerable to the criticisms levelled at Karasek and Theorell's approach. The inclusion of subjective factors means that the model is dependent on self-report data (since no external assessor can objectively determine the perceived degree of reciprocity in effort and rewards), with all of the difficulties this raises (see above). Similarly, the issue of negative affectivity is even more pertinent to the ERI model than it is to the DCS model, because of the focus on subjective feelings at work. How is it possible to disentangle the degree to which perceived lack of reciprocity in effort and rewards is determined by work-related factors, factors outside work, or the elusive personality trait of negative affectivity? By raising questions about the subjective life of the worker, the ERI model reveals the epidemiological fallacy of assuming that a pathogenic agent (job stressors) can be separated from characteristics of the host (other life experiences and affective states/dispositions). There is a circularity in the argument that adverse experiences at work cause negative feelings, but negative feelings lead to negative assessments of work characteristics.

The complex interplay between experiences at work and the worker's attempt to interpret and give meaning to such experiences does not fit well with the linear cause and effect logic of the epidemiological imagination and belies the claim that such processes can be adequately grasped by quantitative methods of inquiry. The difficulty is illustrated in a qualitative study of the health-related experiences of employees in small enterprises. Adopting a 'social interactionist' approach, Eakin and MacEachen[120] found that particular features of working life in small workplaces, especially their personalized social relations and low polarization of employer–employee interests, shaped workers' perceptions of work and its relationship to health. Health problems could be created, aggravated and made chronic through the meanings associated with certain conditions of work, social relations and bodily circumstances. Thus, employees who perceived their employer in negative terms reported quite different health-related experiences to those who enjoyed good relations with the boss; the former were more likely to inflate the severity of health problems and to blame them on work. Eakin and MacEachen conclude:

> The study also underscores the extent to which health status does not exist independently of its subjective interpretation by those experiencing them, and the ways in which this interpretation is bounded by the social relations in which it is embedded.[121]

Siegrist's ERI model nominally recognizes the importance of the subjective processes of interpretation identified by Eakin and MacEachen, but tries to accommodate them within a recognizably epidemiological framework and methodology by reducing them to a small number of quantitative variables. Rather than bolstering the epidemiological approach to work stress, Siegrist only succeeds in revealing its shortcomings as a means of accessing and taking account of the rich subjective life of the worker. As such the ERI model represents a point on the intellectual pathway away from epidemiology towards psychological and sociological accounts of the phenomenon.

The psychological approach to work stress

While the epidemiologists have tended to focus on work characteristics as the major determinant of stress, psychologists have focused more on the personal attributes of the worker and the extent to which they influence the appraisal of threats and the ability to cope. Roy Payne[122] (after Lazarus and Folkman)[123] has produced a model which illustrates the role of psychological factors in mediating the relationship between environmental conditions, cognition and perception of a threat and the onset of mental distress and ultimately illness (see Figure 2.1). A major advance on the epidemiological models of job strain is the recognition that objectively similar working conditions may not have the same effect on different workers.

Whether a situation is actually stressful or not depends upon the individual's appraisal:

> For the masochist, being beaten is presumably a pleasure, and for the successful workaholic, another demanding task is merely a welcome challenge. Perception and cognition determine what the world means to us: one person's threat is another's opportunity.[124]

Figure 2.1 Stress as process

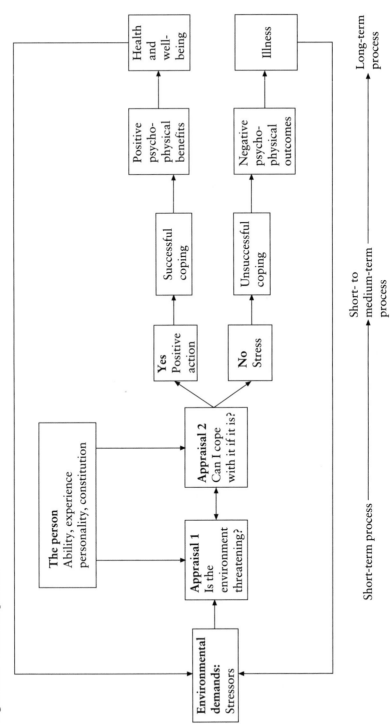

Source: Payne 1999, after Lazarus and Folkman 1984

Appraisal is a two-stage transactional process in which the magnitude of a threat is assessed in comparison with an assessment of the individual's ability to cope with it. Thus, work stress is viewed as a function of the relationship between work characteristics and the attributes of (and resources available to) the individual worker. Primary appraisal of a potential stressor can have three outcomes: it may be deemed irrelevant to the individual concerned, or beneficial ('benign-positive' in Lazarus's parlance), or stressful, i.e. potentially harmful. However, whether a potential stressor actually triggers the stress response depends upon a secondary appraisal of the individual's ability to cope with the potential stressor. This entails a process described as self-efficacy[125] in which questions are asked of oneself, such as 'What choices do I have?'; 'Can I implement a particular option?'; 'Will it work?' A positive appraisal of the capacity to cope with a potential stressor greatly reduces the experience of stress.

Recognition of the role of cognitive appraisal and self-efficacy is a vital advance over epidemiological models of work stress which imply that objective factors in the workplace cause stress and ill health directly irrespective of their interpretation by and meaning for the individual. The process of appraisal explains why some people cope or even thrive in circumstances which others would find unbearably stressful. What then are the factors that influence or determine the appraisal process? Many psychological accounts of work stress have emphasized the role played by personality and its various dimensions.

Perhaps the most basic personality model is that instigated by two cardiologists to explain psychological influences on coronary heart disease. Friedman and Rosenman[126] draw a distinction between people who tend to exhibit Type A behaviour, i.e. ambition, aggressive competitiveness, eagerness to get things done on time, and people who tend to exhibit Type B behaviour which is more relaxed and less competitive. 'Type A man' coincides with lay images of the dynamic corporate executive and the workaholic, pushing the Protestant work ethic to its logical conclusion. The two types can be differentiated through face-to-face interviews or through a self-report questionnaire. It is argued that those exhibiting Type A behaviour are more likely to select themselves into demanding jobs, but are also more likely to over-react to them and are, therefore, more vulnerable to stress and coronary heart disease in particular.

During the 1960s the behaviour types identified by the cardiologists were further explored by psychologists who attempted to identify and measure more precisely the dimensions of the Type A 'personality'.[127] The focus on personality implies that Type A behaviour is something that inheres in the individual as an intrinsic quality or disposition which is largely independent from social and economic relations. There is some evidence to suggest that it is a relatively stable characteristic and it has been demonstrated that Type A and Type B personalities can be differentiated in young children. However,

Riska[128] suggests that efforts to measure the psychological dimensions of the coronary-prone personality only served to fragment the concept leading to a decline in the academic use of the construct in the late 1990s. Certainly, the empirical evidence is mixed; while the British Regional Heart Study found no evidence to support the claim that Type A behaviour predicts major CHD events in middle-aged men,[129] a more recent review by one of the originators of the concept is supportive of a relationship between Type A behaviour and ill health.[130]

One of the difficulties is that Type A behaviour is claimed to be most prevalent among high achievers. Helman even suggests that it is a 'culture-bound syndrome of middle-aged, middle-class men',[131] but, as the Whitehall study indicates, the social gradient for heart disease runs the other way, with greater prevalence among junior grade civil servants. As one commentator has remarked, 'It is not the bosses but the people who are bossed about who suffer most from work stress.'[132] While the conceptual and empirical basis of the Type A thesis may be questionable, its identification of 'executive' stress has had a major impact on lay theories of 'coronary candidacy',[133] and on the public discourse of work stress generally. Moreover, the suggestion that work stress is to be found among those who most vigorously pursue the Protestant work ethic has served to valorize the phenomenon and provide the basis for self-exonerative moral reasoning and claim making on the part of those who occupy positions of power in social and economic hierarchies.

At the height of the British Empire Rudyard Kipling urged potential Victorian imperialists to take up the 'the white man's burden', suggesting that the exploitation and oppression of their colonial subjects was an onerous duty that they should shoulder in order to advance the cause of 'civilization'. A century later the 'burden' of office is more likely to be morally justified by claims that the exercise of power and influence is a cause of work stress. Anecdotal evidence for this observation came from a conversation between one of the authors and a senior civil servant who had recently been obliged to inform a number of junior staff that they were about to be made redundant. Being of a liberal persuasion the senior civil servant had experienced a high degree of anxiety over the incident; however, this anxiety was not expressed as guilt, but as work stress, generated by the strain of executive decision making. As the archetypal headmaster reputedly said before wielding the stick, 'This is going to hurt me far more than you.' The point is not that the anxiety experienced by the civil servant was unreal, but that it was used to reverse the moral status of victim and aggressor. The insecurity and powerlessness of the junior staff who faced losing their livelihood pales before the 'stress' endured by the person exercising power over them.

In contrast with the claims made for Type A behaviour, a second approach to linking personality traits to work stress has focused on an alleged disposition to believe that the main aspects of everyday life are beyond one's control. This fatalistic disposition is described as having an 'external locus of control'.[134] There is evidence to suggest that 'externals' are more likely to become depressed than less fatalistic people who are deemed to have an 'internal locus of control'.[135] It has also been suggested that 'externals' are more likely to respond to perceived stressors with negative emotions or even aggressive behaviour.[136] As with negative affectivity (discussed above), external locus of control may have a strong influence on the appraisal of work characteristics, particularly job control,[137] and confound the apparent relationship between such characteristics and illness.

The fundamental problem with the locus of control thesis is the same as that for Type A behaviour, negative affectivity and other so-called dispositional attributes, such as 'hardiness'[138] or 'sense of coherence';[139] how can these putative personality traits which supposedly cause or exacerbate work stress be distinguished from emotional states which might themselves be caused by experiences at work? Workers in low-grade jobs may well exhibit an external locus of control; however, rather than being an autonomous personality trait this may represent a very astute and rational assessment of the degree of control they have over their lives relative to their more affluent contemporaries. Similarly, the aggressively competitive behaviour of the Type A personality may be a rational response to the incentives and pressures of the traditional middle-class career. It is not sufficient to suggest that this question can be answered by observing that personality traits are stable over time, because exposure to low job control, for instance, can also extend over large sections of the life course and may be a continuation of working-class experiences of low control at school. The point is not that emotional states such as negative affectivity and external locus of control are not real, but that their interpretation as ahistorical autonomous personality traits amounts to a reification of social relations in which the emotional correlates of social experiences (which are structured by factors such as race, gender and class) are detached from their social and economic context. Causality can then be turned on its head, with dispositional attributes used to explain negative appraisals of social experiences (at work and beyond) rather than vice versa.

Not all psychological attempts to explain the extent to which personal attributes influence the appraisal of potential stressors focus on personality traits or types; for example, attention has been paid to coping styles and to external resources such as social support.

As with the concept of cognitive appraisal much of the research on coping has been done by the University of California Berkeley Stress and Coping project led by Richard Lazarus.[140] Again, coping is examined from a cognitive, rather than situational, perspective – one employs cognitive and behavioural efforts to cope, rather than being in a socio-economic position that enables one to cope. A distinction has been drawn between 'problem-focused' and 'emotion-focused' coping styles.[141] The former involves using social skills to arrive at a practical solution to the problem. Emotion-focused coping by contrast involves controlling the emotional response to a stressor, for example by avoidance or denial, or by humour.[142] The suggestion is that problem-focused coping strategies are better than those which are emotion-focused; certainly some emotion-focused strategies, such as smoking tobacco or consuming alcohol or other drugs, may have adverse health consequences of their own, and avoidance and denial may be construed as 'running away' from the problem. Although, as Lazarus has suggested, a little illusion is necessary for good mental health.[143]

Some of the literature on coping styles emphasizes affective dispositions or personality, but others have viewed coping as internal resources which can be learned or modified. Relatively little attention has been paid to the extent to which these internal coping resources are determined or complemented by access to external resources like education and money. An important exception to this is the substantial body of research into the role of social support in mediating the stress response.

For psychologists social support refers to the resources (both emotional and practical) that are derived from an individual's social network of family friends, co-workers and other social contacts. There is a substantial body of empirical evidence suggesting that loneliness, or lack of social support, may lead to ill health, for example Lynch[144] found higher death rates from heart disease among people who were widowed, divorced and never married than among married people. Similarly, Berkman and Syme,[145] in their study of Alameda County residents, found a relationship between social ties (marital status, contacts with family and friends, church membership, and group associations) and mortality from all causes and from a number of specific diseases such as cancer and heart disease. But what is the mechanism by which social support influences health?

There are two dominant models. First it has been suggested that social support brings health benefits irrespective of the degree of stress encountered by the individual; this is the 'main effect model'.[146] A second model suggests that social support acts as a 'buffer' against the negative effects of stress by fulfilling specific needs, through practical help, advice and information or emotional comfort.[147] In fact, the two models are not incompatible. It may well be that social support meets emotional and practical needs throughout the life course, but is particularly beneficial when particular challenges or difficulties arise.

It is useful to conceptualize the different aspects of social support in relationship to the two-stage model of appraisal discussed above. Emotional support in the form of self-esteem enhancing positive regard from others may increase individuals' confidence in their ability to deal with the challenges that confront them, enhancing their perceptions of control and sense of cohesion. Information support may yield new strategies for resolving particular problems, or reduce the perceived magnitude of the challenge by placing it in the context of difficulties encountered by others. Finally, practical or instrumental support may offer the resources to resolve a problem or stop it arising in the first place; for example, the anxiety that may arise from leaving work early to collect children from school might not arise if the burden can be shared with a partner, and the burden of student debt may be eased by affluent and generous parents. Thus, when it comes to appraising a potential stressor, the availability of emotional, information and instrumental support may substantially effect an individual's perception of threat.

While good-quality social support may benefit the individual it necessarily involves entering into a network of social relations that may also have negative effects. First, a large social network exposes the individual to the problems and anxieties of others which may trigger an adverse reaction if the relationship is intimate.[148] Similarly, social relations tend to demand a high degree of reciprocity, so support from others may lead to the burden of providing support for others, which those with limited resources may have difficulty meeting. Moreover, social ties can damage self-esteem as well as enhancing it, not just through interpersonal conflict, but through over-dependence on particular individuals and vulnerability to losing their support, either because it is withdrawn or through bereavement. Particular difficulties may arise when social support is provided by a professional carer, such as a counsellor or general practitioner (see Chapter 5).

The importance of the social support literature lies in the extent to which it reveals that our identity, self-esteem, confidence and coping skills are heavily dependent upon the network of social relations that we enter into and that these relations, therefore, play a key role in the appraisal of potential stressors and the availability of resources for tackling them. This is a much more dynamic conceptualization of the factors that shape the appraisal process than that which is offered by explanations based on personality traits or types. However, the social support literature is based upon a very limited definition of social relations that does not extend beyond direct contact with members of the immediate social network, such as family, friends and work colleagues. In fact we enter into a much broader series of social relations; for instance, through the institutions of the state we enter into relationships with welfare and health care professionals, schoolteachers, and other government representatives, and through the market mechanism we enter into indirect relations with an even broader host of people who produce and distribute other goods and services.

This broader network of social relations may provide emotional, information and instrumental support which has just as much bearing on the appraisal of stressors as the more intimate relations of the immediate social network. For example, the threat of redundancy may be appraised as less of a threat in a society with a low rate of unemployment which offers adequate unemployment benefits and opportunities to retrain than one in which none of these benefits are available. Moreover, this broader social network gives rise to cultural themes and narratives which may also influence an individual's appraisal of the threat posed by potential stressors and his or her ability to overcome them. As we saw in Chapter 1, there exists a public discourse of work stress which may influence the ways in which individuals interpret the threat posed to them by particular experiences at work and their ability to cope with such experiences.

The extent to which experiences, perceptions and interpretations of work stress are influenced by broader social and cultural influences will be explored in Chapter 4. For now it is sufficient to recognize that the insights offered by psychological accounts of the work stress phenomenon are constrained by the discipline's focus on the individual's attributes and immediate milieu.

The individualizing tendency of the psychological discourse of work stress is apparent in the Person–Environment Fit Model (PEF) which suggests that stress occurs when there is either a real or perceived mismatch between the demands/stressors in a particular environment (say a job) and the knowledge, skills, abilities and needs of the person.[149–151] Few would argue with the wisdom of ensuring that workers are not placed in jobs which they lack the resources to cope with, and, by definition, the model captures the relationship between environmental and personal factors, implying that the modification of job characteristics to suit the individual is just as viable as modifying or selecting individuals to suit the job. In practice, however, employers may be more likely to focus on the latter strategy, either by administering psychometric tests to individuals prior to recruitment, or by teaching stress management skills to those already employed:

> The usual assumption of individually tailored interventions based on such a model is that increasing a person's knowledge and skills will offset the impact of stressors in the workplace through improved coping resources. As a result many of the techniques used to effect change are based on personality and coping models.[152]

As the above observation implies, the assumption is that the factors which shape the individual can be reduced to personality traits or coping skills, and that the appropriate point of intervention is, therefore, the individual worker. However, as the analysis presented above suggests, the appraisal process may be significantly shaped both by broader cultural norms and crucially by the individual's location in a broad network of social relations which confer varying degrees of access to material, cultural and emotional resources. By dichotomizing the person and environment the PEF effectively denies the social character of the appraisal process, leading to a narrow focus on individualized solutions.

A strong reinforcement of psychology's individualized approach to the work stress phenomenon is the evidence that stress can be conceptualized as physiological arousal which may have consequences for health, and it is to the physiology of stress that we now turn.

Physiological accounts of stress

Both the public and scientific discourses of work stress depend on the claim that our thoughts and feelings can have such a powerful impact on the physiology of the body that they can cause severe illness and death. Such a proposition runs counter to one of the central tenets of western philosophy (most famously expounded by Descartes,[153] but traceable back to Anaxagorous); that mind and body are fundamentally different substances, that the body is ultimately little more than a mechanical device, governed by the laws of physics, but that the mind or soul is a different substance capable of thought, free will and essentially beyond the reach of scientific laws. But how can a substance as apparently ethereal as the mind have an influence on physiology? Descartes' answer to the mind–body problem focused on the pineal gland which he saw as the physical site of interaction between the body and the soul, through which the soul could both direct the body and be affected by physical stimuli.[154] Descartes' formulation was unsatisfactory even to his followers and modern physiologists have attempted to transcend the problems of Cartesian dualism by adopting a materialist account of emotions and their impact on the body, in which the stress response figures prominently. Materialism dispenses with dualism in favour of the belief that mental life is essentially physical, i.e. that it is explicable in terms of the combinations of matter in movement. However, as we shall see, despite this detailed mapping of the stressed body physiologists have failed to provide a satisfactory account of the extent to which stress is mediated by consciousness.

The body's response to stress is governed by a complex series of interactions between the nervous system and the endocrine system. The nervous system is like a telephone network, comprising neural fibres that run through the body connecting organs and converging in the brain. The endocrine system is more like a postal service made up of glands throughout the body which communicate with organs by releasing specially addressed hormones into the blood stream, rather than through direct wired connections. Thus,

> information can be transmitted as fast, but short-lasting messages through the nervous system, or it can be transmitted as slow, but long-lasting messages through the endocrine system.[155]

Key to the stress response is part of the brain located just above the roof of the mouth called the hypothalamus which governs basic bodily functions, such as eating, sleeping, sexuality and strong emotions, sometimes referred to as the four Fs (fighting, fleeing, feeding and mating). Once a threat has been recognized the hypothalamus initiates the physiological changes that prepare the body for action by acting on the autonomic nervous system (ANS) and the endocrine system. The ANS, as its name suggests, is relatively independent from the central nervous system (brain and spinal cord) and has two subdivisions called the sympathetic and parasympathetic nervous systems.

The sympathetic system brings about the state of high arousal first described by Walter Cannon as the fight or flight response (see above). These physiological changes are triggered by the release of the hormones epinephrine (adrenaline) and norepinephrine (noradrenaline) from the medulla or core of the adrenal glands. The parasympathetic system reverses the changes brought about by the sympathetic system, returning the body to a state of homeostasis and promoting energy conservation.

The hypothalamus also acts on the endocrine system by stimulating the pituitary gland to release adrenocorticotrophic hormone (ACTH) into the blood stream, which in turn causes the adrenal cortex (the outer part of the adrenal glands) to swell and release hormones. In terms of the stress response the most important group of hormones secreted by the adrenal cortex is the glucocorticoids which regulate blood glucose levels, blood pressure, inflammation and immune reactions. Cortisol is one of the major glucocorticoids and is often cited as one of the 'stress hormones'.

The autonomic nervous system and the endocrine system are the communication systems through which the brain prepares the body for action; however, the flow of information is not just in one direction. There is a neural feedback loop from the adrenal glands to the hypothalamus (via the hippocampus) which transmits information about adrenal function back to the brain. Similarly, although almost all pituitary hormones are governed by the hypothalamus, they not only act upon bodily systems but are also carried to the brain as neuropeptides where they play a major role in the regulation of brain function.

Although physiologists have mapped the mechanisms by which the brain activates the physiological changes that comprise the stress response they have still not resolved the mind–body problem that vexed Descartes. The actions of the hypothalamus on the autonomic nervous system and endocrine system are well documented, but what role does conscious thought play in the process? The key role of the autonomic nervous system implies that the stress response is largely beyond conscious control, but the hypothalamus must in some way be responding to external stimuli, i.e. it must be responding to a perceived threat. The answer lies in the relationship between the limbic system (of which the hypothalamus is a part) which regulates emotions and aspects of physiology, and the systems of the brain that control consciousness and thought. As early as the 1930s it was recognized that the linkage between these systems was poor:[156]

The limbic system is most centrally involved in emotions and related physiological reactions, but is not strongly connected to the system that controls thought and language. Our inability to do what we think we should do or to feel what we prefer to feel is based on this relative skimpiness of linkages between these systems. [157]

But what form does the skimpiness of this neural linkage take and what does it tell us about the pathway from perception of an external threat through to the triggering of the stress response? A metaphor for this relationship might be two separate conversations taking place in adjacent rooms. If the discussants in each room listen carefully they can hear what is being said next door, but their ability to influence the discussion is extremely limited. Following this metaphor, it may be that the hypothalamus or other parts of the limbic system 'overhear a conversation' about the magnitude of a potential stressor that is taking place in the part of the brain that controls language and thought. This might explain the process by which the cognitive process of appraisal described by the psychologists (see above) triggers the stress response – although, of course, rather than being an actual conversation that is overheard, it is the activity of neurons in one part of the brain that is being weakly transmitted to the limbic system. By the same process, information about the physiological changes in the body that accompany the stress response may also be transmitted back into consciousness.

Alternatively it has been suggested by Siegrist[158] (after LeDoux)[159] that the pathway from chronic exposure to an unfavourable psycho-social work environment through to the physiological stress response is 'largely independent of cognitive information processing', and that, therefore, 'many workers doing the same job over a longer period may feel distressed and aroused even though they do not exactly know why'.

Certainly, in subjective terms the fight or flight response often seems to be triggered before a potential threat has been subjected to a rational process of appraisal. Also, the stress response may be quite irrational, for instance in the case of phobias. In such instances the limbic system seems to override the rational appraisal process, and one may be conscious of struggling with one's emotions by trying to impose a rational appraisal of non-threat onto a body that is responding as if life itself is threatened. But how can the pathway from perception of external stimuli be presented to the limbic system as a threat without the mediation of consciousness? One possibility is that the recognition of certain stimuli as a threat to the organism is 'hard-wired' into the brain as an instinctive response determined by evolutionary pressures. This might explain some of the phobias; for instance, a predisposition to run away from spiders and snakes may have been of immense adaptive value to our ancestors, but it surely cannot explain why more recent threats, such as those associated with adverse work characteristics, should be able to short-cut conscious appraisal and automatically trigger the stress response.

An alternative solution might be that such responses are learned or conditioned across the life course and that they become so deeply embedded in our psychological make-up that they can trigger the stress response without reference to (or even in opposition to) conscious appraisal. Readers will be familiar with the classic studies conducted by Pavlov which demonstrated how dogs could be conditioned to associate food with the ringing of a bell, and subsequently to salivate when the bell was rung in the absence of food.[160] Similarly, there is evidence that the immune system can be conditioned to respond in the absence of an antigen (see below). Perhaps then the stress response can be conditioned to respond reflexively to particular external stimuli without conscious mediation. The process by which social experiences become embedded in the body over the life course is explored in the next chapter; for now it is sufficient to note that this question is substantially a psycho-social one to which physiological accounts of the stress response have not yet provided a satisfactory answer.

As well as describing the biological processes that comprise the fight or flight response, physiologists have also attempted to plot the pathway between stress and illness. We have already briefly noted the role of Hans Selye's General Adaptation Syndrome (GAS) in the pathologization of the stress response (see above). The GAS is a three-stage model which explores the physiological changes that occur if the high levels of arousal that characterize the fight or flight response are maintained over a long period of time, rather than subsiding as an acute stressor is dealt with and the parasympathetic nervous system returns the body to a state of homeostasis. The secretion of ACTH from the pituitary gland and its subsequent effect of swelling the adrenal cortex leading to the release of cortisol (among other hormones) plays a central role in the GAS. If arousal is maintained through the stages of alarm and resistance and into the final stage of exhaustion, then the increased levels of cortisol will adversely effect the immune, digestive, circulatory and other bodily systems, ultimately resulting in the death of the organism.

Selye claimed that the stress response was non-specific, that is that essentially the same response would occur whatever the stressor, be it physical or psychological. However, this claim fails to take adequate account of the influence of psycho-social factors. Thus, the strength of the emotional response triggered by a particular stressor influences the endocrinological response, and although particular emotional states cannot be matched precisely to specific patterns of neurohormonal reactivity, there is evidence that different patterns of endocrine activity are broadly related to particular emotional states – for example, anger appears to be associated with increased noradrenaline, while fear is associated with higher levels of adrenaline.[161] Similarly, it is generally the case that the stronger the emotional response the greater the production of cortisol, adrenaline and noradrenaline.[162] Despite these criticisms of Selye's initial formulation of the GAS, the broader claim that the physiological changes which comprise the stress response can, if sufficiently prolonged, lead to pathological changes is supported by a substantial body of empirical evidence.

Much of this evidence comes from primate studies. Richard Sapolsky's work with wild male baboons in the Serengeti has proven particularly influential.[163–4] Baboons spend just four hours per day meeting their food requirements, leaving at least twelve hours for social interaction. As a result they have an extensive and hierarchical social network in which dominant baboons have greater rights to grooming and sexual behaviour than subordinate baboons, enforced by stand-offs and minor scuffles. Examination revealed the effects of these patterns of dominance on the physiology of the subordinate baboons. Not only did they have more bite marks, they also had a greater prevalence of stomach ulcers and higher levels of glucocorticoids in their blood, which Sapolsky demonstrated was attributable to the stress associated with their subordinate position in the social hierarchy.

Further evidence shows that not only do low-status primates have higher levels of cortisol (one of the glucocorticoids associated with the stress response), but that continued exposure reduces the effectiveness of the feedback mechanism between the adrenals and the hypothalamus by causing a degeneration of the receptors in the hippocampus, leading to higher basal rates of cortisol even when the animal is not directly exposed to a stressor.[165–7] The hippocampus also plays a role in memory and it has been suggested that memory loss in old age may result from exposure to chronic stress earlier in the life course. In addition to raised levels of glucocorticoids, Sapolsky also found physiological changes which would be considered risk factors for cardiovascular disease in humans. Low-status baboons had higher blood pressure than the dominant apes, which was slower to reduce after a stressful incident and had a higher basal rate. Similarly, the high cortisol levels found in the low-status baboons was associated with higher levels of high-density lipoproteins (HDL – which can lead to faster build-up of cholesterol deposits in the arteries), and lower levels of low-density lipoproteins (LDL – which help to clear the arteries). The lowered HDL/LDL ratio was associated with narrowing of the coronary artery and aorta in low-status animals.

One criticism of Sapolsky's findings might be that they were attributable to social selection, i.e. that less healthy animals were less able to compete and, therefore, ended up at the bottom of the social hierarchy. However, Sapolsky demonstrated that glucocorticoid levels changed when an ape left its original group and took on a new social status in a different group, suggesting that the changes were attributable to psycho-social stress rather than selection.

Although Sapolsky's work is convincing, questions remain about the extent to which it is possible to generalize from animal studies to humans, not just because of physiological differences, but because of the obvious cognitive and behavioural differences. The stress encountered by Sapolsky's apes literally involved fight or flight as subordinate baboons were faced down by dominant rivals. While aggressive exchanges in the human workplace are not unheard of, work stress is usually taken to refer to less confrontational aspects of the psycho-social environment, such as heavy workload, or job insecurity. Are such stressors likely to provoke the same physiological responses in humans that occur in stressed animals? And are such changes of functional importance?

Before leaving Sapolsky's work, it is worth noting his observation about the history of human anatomy, which suggests that humans may endure a similar response to animals. During the century from 1830 nearly all of the bodies used to teach anatomy in London medical schools were obtained from the city's poorhouses. The adrenal glands of the corpses tended to be much larger than would be considered normal today. When the anatomists occasionally saw the adrenals of a more affluent corpse, they were often found to be much smaller and a new disease – *idiopathic adrenal atrophy* – was invented to explain it. Not until the twentieth century was it recognized that the small adrenals of the rich were actually normal and that those of the poor had been enlarged by their prolonged exposure to socio-economic stress. Similarly, the shrunken thymus glands of the poor were also taken for the 'norm' and the larger thymus of rich patients were classed as a disorder and treated with radiation therapy which often led to thyroid cancer.[168] Although indicative of a link between stress and physiological changes in humans, Sapolsky's historical observation is far from conclusive. However, there is also more compelling physiological evidence, particularly concerning immune function and cardiovascular disease. Two relatively 'new' disciplines, psychoneuroimmunology and econeurocardiology, have attempted to map the relationship between external stimuli, the stress response and, respectively, immune function and cardiovascular disease. First we will consider the contribution of psychoneuroimmunology.

Psychoneuroimmunology (PNI)

A number of studies on humans suggests that psycho-social stress may play a role in reducing the effectiveness of the immune system. One of the more convincing examples was a blind randomized controlled trial conducted by Cohen *et al.*[169] Volunteers were asked to complete a questionnaire to measure their stress levels and were then randomly assigned to two groups. Nasal drops containing a range of cold viruses were administered to the experimental group, while the control group were given nasal drops that were virus-free. Twenty-seven per cent of subjects with a low-stress rating went on to develop a cold, compared with 47 per cent of those with a high-stress rating. The association remained even after controlling for gender, educational attainment, allergic status, alcohol and tobacco consumption, exercise, diet and sleep loss. Other experiments have produced similar findings; for instance, medical students were found to have suppressed immune function (reduced T-cell and NK cell counts) during stressful exams.[170-2] Similarly, residents exposed to the anxiety of living near to the Three Mile Island nuclear plant (in the years following the accident that occurred there) were found to have suppressed immune function compared to control groups living further away.[173]

Not all of the evidence has supported the relationship between psycho-social factors and immune dysfunction, and the functional significance of such changes has also been questioned, although the equivocal nature of some of the published data may be attributable to issues around the use and interpretation of *in vitro* and *in vivo* immunological and virological assays.[174] Some studies even suggest that immune function may be enhanced by brief exposure to stressors. Volunteers who were asked to complete mental arithmetic questions to the accompaniment of loud music showed transient increases in the number of suppressor/cytotoxic T-lymphocytes and natural killer cell activity, and parachutists making their first descent were found to have an increase in the number and activity of their natural killer cells.[175] Similarly, mice exposed to noise stress over a five and a half week period exhibited a drop in immune function during the first few weeks (a drop in the responsiveness and cell-killing ability of B- and T-lymphocytes), followed by an increase in immune function to beyond that found in unstressed mice, before eventually returning to normal.[176] Variations in immune function over the duration of a chronic stressor reveal the complexity of the relationship between the immune system and the different physiological changes that comprise the stress response. Moreover, there is a question of whether the positive or negative effect of a potential stressor on the immune function is in any way influenced by what the individual makes of the stressor subjectively.

The physiological changes which accompany the stress response appear to have a number of effects on vital components of the immune system. ACTH lowers the production of antibodies; the glucocorticoids reduce immune cell activity and reduce the number of lymphocytes; and epinephrine influences lymphocyte metabolism.[177] Moreover, there is anatomical evidence of interconnections between the central nervous system (CNS) and key components of the immune system such as the thymus[178] and the lymphoid tissue.[179] Similarly, receptors for particular neurotransmitters and hormones have been found on the surface of immune cells, for example B-adrenoreceptors in T- and B-lymphocytes.[180–1] This evidence of an apparent link between the CNS and the immune system lies behind the basic question of PNI:

> If the brain is capable of exerting some influence on the modulation of immune responses, can the CNS convey the effects of psycho-social factors on a variety of immunologically mediated pathophysiological processes?[182]

Despite the growing evidence to support the PNI thesis there remains a reluctance among related disciplines to accept that the immune system can be affected by psycho-social factors.[183] A key problem may be that of conceptualizing how the relationship between brain and immune system is mediated; for example, does consciousness play a role? One of the pathways between external stimuli and immune response appears to be largely autonomic. Robert Ader, for many the founding father of PNI, demonstrated that immune response could be conditioned in rats in the same way that Pavlov's dogs could be conditioned to salivate.[184] Ader used classical conditioning techniques to establish a link between the taste of saccharin solution and the immune suppressing action of cyclophosphomide, so that immune suppression continued to occur when saccharin solution was administered even when the cyclophosphomide had been withdrawn. Further studies have confirmed Ader's findings.

A similar experiment, this time on guinea pigs, has demonstrated that activation of the immune system can also be classically conditioned. Dwyer's experiment involved the grafting of rabbit skin onto the backs of the guinea pigs, thus provoking the immune response to reject the foreign tissue. The grafts were repeated and each time they were accompanied by other stimuli such as bright lights, loud music, injection of local anaesthetic and heavy bandaging after the transplant. This procedure was repeated three times, but on the third replication no rabbit skin was actually transplanted, although all the other stimuli were present. Dwyer found that although there was no rabbit skin present for the guinea pigs' immune system to reject, biopsy of the area where the skin would have been revealed highly active t-cells searching for the 'expected' graft.[185]

Thus, the link between psycho-social stimuli and the immune response may be either a by-product of the endocrine activity that accompanies the stress response, or the result of largely unconscious learned or conditioned responses. It has also been hypothesized that genetic factors may influence neuroendocrine-immune interactions, although little research has yet been done on this.[186] But to what extent can changes in immune function be governed by conscious thought? We will return to this question after considering evidence of the relationship between psycho-social stimuli and health derived from another relatively new discipline – econeurocardiology.

Econeurocardiology (ENC)

That emotional experiences can have an effect on the heart has long been a common theme in western culture, but science has adopted a much more equivocal stance on the question of 'heartbreak'. The role of the forebrain in cardiovascular regulation was reported by Rene Leriche as early as 1931,[187-8] yet these neuroregulatory mechanisms continue to be overlooked by most medical textbooks, which it has been suggested reflects the 'pedagogic error' of subdividing the teaching of medical students into clinical specialties.[189] The field developed rapidly from the 1970s onwards, with the development of a new subdiscipline – econeurocardiology[190] – which focuses on the relationship between environmental stimuli, the nervous system and cardiovascular development and disease. These 'environmental stimuli' often stem from our relations with others, particularly when a threat is encountered, although other factors that stimulate a strong emotional response are also included.

Several sites in the forebrain have been implicated in cardiovascular regulation through the autonomic processes and via direct neural pathways to the heart: the insular cortex, hypothalamus, medial frontal cortex, septum, thalamus, zona incerta, amygdala, and bed nuclea of the stria terminalis.[191] The neurological pathway from environmental stimuli to the cardiovascular system is responsible for a wide range of bodily effects, from blushing in response to an embarrassing comment through to sudden death, for instance in the case of voodoo death in Central America, and Pouri Pouri in the Pacific Islands.[192] But what are the mechanisms by which emotional responses can damage the heart?

It has been suggested that chronic exposure to stressors can result in 'hyperfunctional overdrive', that is, over-stimulation by the catecholamine system, which brings about a 'constant state of visceral-vascular readiness'.[193] Catecholamine excess can create cardiac electrical instability resulting in sudden arrhythmic death (the most common mode of death among adults under 65 in industrialized countries).[194] Belkic[195] suggests three mechanisms by which catecholamine excess can invoke tachyarrhythmias: increased automatic activity (increased slope of Phase 4 depolarization and in slow inward calcium current in partially depolarized cells; augmented early and late triggering (facilitation of calcium influx); re-entry (lowered Phase 4 potential slows conduction, increases internal resistance, and diminishes cell-to-cell conduction, which promotes asynchronous repolarization).

The stress response is also implicated in the development of atherosclerosis (the formation of lesions and fibrous plaques on the arterial wall). Evidence of the mechanisms behind this process from human studies is inconsistent, although hypertension, the production of Angiotensin II, and a high LDL/HDL ratio play a role and may be influenced by stress.[196] Fibrinogen has also been linked with work stress and contributes to coronary heart disease through its role in atherosclerosis and clot formation.[197]

The pathways between activation of the autonomic nervous system, the hypothalamic–pituitary–adrenal axis, and immune function/cardiovascular health have been reliably mapped. However, the functional significance of particular physiological changes and the reliability and validity of assaying such changes is not clearly understood; for example, what constitutes a dangerously high level of fibrinogen or catecholamines, and can variations in levels be solely attributed to the stress response? These questions remain largely unanswered and therefore undermine the significance of studies which have demonstrated an association between environmental stimuli (such as work characteristics) and raised levels of various 'stress' hormones. Job strain may be associated with raised fibrinogen levels (among other changes), but whether such changes are sufficient to effect cardiovascular disease remains unclear.

Moreover, despite their prefixs, *psycho*neuroimmunology and *eco*neurocardiology have tended to focus on mapping the neurological pathways between the brain and immune function/the cardiovascular system, and have not addressed the processes by which the relationship between external stimuli and the physiology of the stress response are mediated by consciousness or, conversely, the effects that these physiological changes have on conscious thought. As the following quotation from a leading econeurocardiologist illustrates, the symbolic character of stressors and the voluntary (or willed) nature of the response is recognized:

> Bodily responses triggered by a thought or by a perception of one's surroundings are attributable, of course, to symbolic as contrasted with tangible stimuli. The bodily changes observed constitute a part of the behaviour of a person, behaviour that is governed by the significance of the situation to the implicated individual. There is, indeed, a vast repertoire of behaviours that adapt the individual to life experiences of all sorts. Each involves discrete patterned responses that are activated and coordinated by the nervous system, and may involve voluntary as well as involuntary behaviour.[198]

The symbolic, semantic, willed component of the eco-neuro-cardio pathway (and of the psycho-neuro-immune pathway) represents the limits of the physiological approach to stress. We know from the psychologists that the appraisal process (as it is influenced by factors such as negative affectivity, locus of control, coping skills, social support, and a host of other psychosocial experiences) plays an important role in mediating the relationship between external stimuli and the physiology of the stress response. The appraisal process must have a material form, i.e. it must exist as patterns of neuro-electro-chemical activity, but, apart from using brain scans to illustrate which parts of the brain are active, for example when we speak, neurologists are not able to give a satisfactory account of how and why we think as we do. Thus, an econeurocardiologist and a psychoneuroimmunologist could no more explain how a brain appraises a stimulus as stressful than they could explain how someone falls in love. All that can be done is to assay the physiological changes that *result* from such an appraisal. In short, PNI and ENC have not resolved the mind–body problem.

Summary

In the first half of this chapter evidence was presented of the extent to which, over its relatively brief history, the scientific discourse of work stress has been influenced by the political, economic and social concerns of the times in which it was produced. From the Social Darwinism and eugenics of the pre-war period, through the military–industrial concerns of cold war America, and the workers' democracy movement in Northern Europe, work stress has provided a medium through which these sometimes contradictory concerns could be articulated and legitimated. However, this does not necessarily mean that all the scientific evidence concerning work stress is purely fictional, and in the second half of the chapter the strengths and weaknesses of contemporary epidemiological, psychological and physiological accounts were appraised.

The first point to note is the relatively poor fit between the lay discourse of work stress described in the first chapter and the scientific evidence presented above. While many themes which occur in the scientific discourse of work stress can also be found in the lay discourse, the evidence is often used selectively, methodological and conceptual difficulties are frequently ignored, and the subsequent claims and conclusions often go beyond the evidence. The lay discourse unquestioningly states that work stress is of epidemic proportions, yet although epidemiologists have attempted to produce a reliable prevalence rate, their findings are questionable on methodological and conceptual grounds. Similarly, work stress (defined in terms of a wide range of work-related experiences) is often cited as a cause of a vast number of illnesses, yet although there is epidemiological evidence of associations between certain work characteristics and particular diseases, and plausible physiological pathways in between, evidence of the exposure required to produce illness and the role of mediating factors is far from conclusive. Most importantly, the lay discourse of work stress is heavily influenced by the disease model employed by epidemiology, and tends to overlook the role of personal attributes and subjectivity.

A second point which emerges from consideration of the different disciplinary approaches to work stress is the extent of the inconsistencies and discontinuities between them. The physiological account of stress in terms of the fight or flight response, endocrine activity etc. may be narrower than the range of experiences which might be self-reported as examples of work stress in epidemiological studies, which may include relatively moderate emotional responses, such as dissatisfaction, impatience, frustration. These relatively minor emotional difficulties may or may not trigger the physiological changes which accompany the fight or flight response, and consequently may or may not give rise to the health problems associated with chronic arousal. This discontinuity between physiological accounts of the stress response and the definitions which inform self-reports of stressful experiences gives rise to the illusion that the relatively mundane trials and tribulations of the working day are likely to give rise to serious pathology.

A similar problem stems from the inability of science to resolve the mind–body problem. Although most contributors to the debate would presumably accept the materialist claim that subjectivity is essentially physical, i.e. residing exclusively in the structures and pathways of the central nervous system, there necessarily remains a latent dualism at the heart of the scientific discourse of work stress. The difficulty resides in the transition from psychological accounts of the appraisal process into physiological accounts of the triggering of the fight or flight response. PNI and ENC often elide this transition, but it actually represents a shift between two fundamentally different modes of explanation.

Psychological accounts of appraisal are concerned with the production of meaning; a process which they explain in terms of a rational evaluation of the scale of a potential threat and the resources available to meet it. This process may be influenced by personality attributes, but it remains an essentially conscious process of interpretation and meaning creation. Physiologists currently have little insight into the bio-mechanics of interpretive processes of this kind. While many may recognize the importance of appraisal in triggering the stress response, they have to take the psychologist's word for it.

This dichotomy between the subjective and physiological dimensions of the stress response masks the overlap between the two. We have noted the extent to which the conscious element of the pathway between external stimuli and the stress response might be short-circuited by classical conditioning and possibly by other mechanisms which create a reflexive response to external stimuli. Hence, the physiological response to a stressor may not always come after a conscious process of appraisal, but before it. An individual may experience an almost instantaneous physical response to a stressor, and this may affect whether or not the stressor is appraised as a threat. Thus, rather than a linear pathway from external stimuli, to cognitive appraisal, to physiological response, we see a much more dynamic and interactive relationship between environment, mind and body.

Some of these interactions may take place unconsciously or autonomically; however, it does seem that consciousness plays an important role in mediating the complex network of interactions between psychosocial stressors and their physiological effects on the body. Thus, individuals faced by a potential threat may feel that they are grappling with their emotions, attempting to persuade themselves that they can cope with the challenge, telling themselves to stay calm, often while struggling to maintain control over the surface of the body, so that the outward signs of anxiety (such as shaking and raised voice pitch) are concealed from others.

It is this inner conversation or struggle that lies at the core of the stress phenomenon. It explains why some people stand up to pressures and demands which others cannot face. It is where our beliefs about courage, bravery and resilience come from, but it is almost entirely overlooked in the public discourse of work stress where, for the most part, stress is treated as an occupational injury that simply befalls individuals exposed to particular experiences at work. One reason for this omission might be that it is seen as victim-blaming, or that it individualizes problems which have situational causes. However, recognizing that resilience resides within the individual and the conscious struggle to cope with a threat or challenge does not mean that the determinants of resilience are not determined by social, economic and cultural factors. In an immediate way resources such as social support may influence perceptions of ability to cope, and cultural norms may affect the importance attached to struggling to cope. However, these external factors also have a less direct effect that develops over the life course, as the body learns (both consciously and unconsciously) how to respond (both physiologically and behaviourally) to perceived threats.

Conceptualizing the interplay of socio-cultural factors, patterns of physiological response and the development of self-identity and resilience over the life course requires a radical departure from epidemiological, psychological and physiological approaches to work stress. In the next chapter we offer an alternative theoretical framework derived from the sociology of the emotions and embodiment. The centrality of consciousness and the production of meaning in the pathway from environmental stressors to the physiological changes associated with the stress response also requires a methodology quite different to the quantitative and experimental techniques of epidemiology, psychology and physiology. Chapter 3, therefore, also contains further evidence from our own qualitative research into the work stress phenomenon.

# 3 Body, self, meaning

In the previous chapter we looked at the contributions to the scientific discourse of work stress that have been made by the disciplines of epidemiology, psychology and physiology. Each of these disciplines has provided very different insights into the work stress phenomenon, but they share a common tendency to understate the mediating role of conscious interpretation and the extent to which the meanings ascribed to adverse experiences at work are shaped by historically specific socio-cultural factors.

This is most clearly the case with the physiological approach to work stress, which, as a subdiscipline of biology, is primarily concerned with measuring the physical structures of the body without recourse to their representation in human consciousness. Essentially physiological disciplines such as psychoneuroimmunology and econeurocardiology have attempted to span or even dispense with the mind–body dichotomy, but for the most part, their appreciation of conscious thought and human emotional life does not extend beyond seeing them as 'input variables' which trigger a series of neuroendocrinological responses.

Despite its concern with environmental and situational influences on the stress response, the social epidemiological perspective on the human subject closely mirrors the materialist perspective of the physiologists. Thus, attempts are made to establish a reliable prevalence rate by counting cases, and to establish statistical relationships between work characteristics and health outcomes, without considering the role played by human consciousness in mediating these relationships and behaviours. Social epidemiologists may have mapped the broad contours of the relationship between work and illness, but they tend to be overly mechanistic, viewing health problems as automatic and unmediated responses to changes in the working environment.

Superficially, the psychological approach to work stress with its emphasis on the process of cognitive appraisal and personality traits would appear to be the antithesis of the reductionist perspective adopted by physiologists and epidemiologists. However, much of the psychological literature on work stress tends to view consciousness in highly individualized and ahistorical terms. This is particularly the case with accounts which focus on the role of personality traits in influencing the appraisal process, for example negative affectivity, external locus of control and the type A personality. Personality traits are often viewed as fixed attributes of the individual (which are often implied to be heavily determined by innate factors), without regard to the way in which these characteristics may develop and change over the life course in response to different social experiences. Social and organizational psychologists have taken account of the way in which individual responses to stress can be influenced by social relations, for example through social support or the adoption of particular roles. However, the psychological conception of social relations rarely extends beyond the individual's immediate milieu or social/kinship network, and it is rare to find a psychological account of work stress which examines the individual's location in a broader web of social, economic and cultural relations; for instance, the influences of race, gender and class are often overlooked. Similarly, changing cultural forms and their influence on consciousness and behaviour are also often overlooked; for example, the question of how individual beliefs and responses are influenced by the public discourse of work stress is rarely asked, even by social psychologists. This rather narrow conception of human consciousness also has methodological consequences. Personality traits are often treated almost as objective characteristics which can be measured and quantified using psychometric tests and then fed into statistical models, for example to predict the extent to which a person 'fits' his or her work environment, or to be controlled for as potential confounding variables in the pathway from work characteristics to illness. Rather less attention is paid to accessing the meanings and definitions which shape the individual's interpretations of social experiences and the ways in which attitudes and beliefs are constantly constructed and negotiated, not just through everyday interaction with friends, relatives and work colleagues, but also through engagement with social and economic institutions and cultural forms.

As we suggested in Chapter 2, the reluctance of psychology to engage fully with the subjective life of the worker has created a lacuna in the pathway from work characteristics to the physiological changes associated with the stress response. The role of consciousness in mediating this relationship is reduced to a rational process of calculation, as the worker appraises the magnitude of a threat and his or her ability to meet it, and the (irrational?) influence of personality traits on this process. But what if the individual's appraisals and reports are shaped by broader social and cultural factors?

As we saw in Chapter 2, Eakin and MacEachen[1] have attempted to address this deficiency by adopting a 'social interactionist' approach which has led them to suggest that health problems can be created, aggravated and made chronic through the meanings associated with certain conditions of work and that these subjective interpretations are bounded by the social relations in which the worker is located. Emphasis is, therefore, shifted towards a more phenomenological approach to understanding the origins of negative feelings about work.

Emphasizing the role of consciousness and broader socio-cultural factors in the work stress phenomenon does not necessarily entail the adoption of a 'pure' social constructionist perspective, or the denial of work stress as a physiologically embodied experience.[2] Recent theoretical developments in the sociology of emotions[3] and embodiment[4] underline the need to conceptualize the stressed worker as an emotionally expressive, embodied subject, who is active in the context of power and social control.[5] Thus, rather than being a passive object of study the worker is transformed into a conscious subject, negotiating his or her relationship to the external world, but also affected by it at both a conscious and physiological level. The strength of adopting an embodied sociological perspective on work stress is that it offers a theoretical framework that is sufficiently broad to incorporate the insights of epidemiology, psychology and physiology; facilitating their synthesis within a broader social, economic and cultural context. But what does an embodied sociology comprise?

Embodied sociology

Since the first edition of Bryan Turner's *Body and Society*[6] was published in 1984 sociological interest in 'the body' has become increasingly overt, with the publication of numerous books on the topic[7-10] and the establishment of a new journal called *Body and Society*, although, as Williams and Bendelow have pointed out, corporeal concerns have always been at the heart of the sociological enterprise, from Marx and Weber, through to Goffman and Bourdieu, even if they have not always been made explicit.[11] Despite this apparent continuity Williams and Bendelow argue that earlier accounts have produced a 'disembodied' sociology of the body, which can be contrasted with the 'new mode of social theorising "from" lived bodies.'[12] Following Frank,[13] the argument is made for an embodied sociology which puts 'minds back in bodies, bodies back into society and society back into the body'. We saw in the previous chapter that attempts to explain the work stress phenomenon in terms of the physiology of the human body have often led to a neglect of the role played by consciousness in mediating the pathway from external stimuli to the stress response – a case of body in, mind out. If an embodied sociology is to avoid this pitfall it must address the mind–body problem. Williams and Bendelow base their assault on the Cartesian dualist legacy substantially on Maurice Merleau-Ponty's phenomenological analysis of the body-subject.[14–17]

Merleau-Ponty's approach to embodiment came from his application of Husserl's phenomenology of intentional consciousness to the corporeal aspects of human existence. From this perspective the Cartesian separation of mind and body is replaced by a non-dualist ontology which posits the 'body-subject' which is always situated in concrete lived experience. Where Descartes drew a distinction between extended substance (matter) and thinking substance (the mind), Merleau-Ponty claimed an irreducible unity between the psychic and the physiological. Thus, perception is not an internal representation of an external world, but a means of being in the world. We observe the world from a particular location or perspective (rather than having a God's eye view), as we directly engage the world through our senses.[18] Merleau-Ponty's analysis of perception suggests that we exist in the world through our bodies and our mode of being is, therefore, irreducibly embodied. Thus, the dichotomy drawn by Descartes between matter in extension and matter which thinks is transcended in Merleau-Ponty's approach.

The embodied perspective also provided Merleau-Ponty with a corporeal basis for understanding intersubjectivity, that is, our awareness that there are other minds in the world. We engage the world through our bodies, but the flow of data is not unidirectional; it is not just the world acting on the individual, but the individual acting on the world (and entering into corporeal relationships with others) through practical activity. The hand that touches can also be touched; the eye that sees can also be seen. It is this reversibility that occurs as we engage in practical activity with others that makes us aware that there are minds in the world other than our own.

The problems with Descartes' dualist approach to the mind–body problem were discussed in the previous chapter and Merleau-Ponty's alternative account of the sentient body-subject clearly represents a route out of the impasse, but does it, as Williams and Bendelow suggest, provide 'the foundation for a truly non-dualist ontology of the body'? Merleau-Ponty was surely correct in adopting a materialist account of consciousness, grounding human thought in the firing of neurons and other physiological processes, rather than in religious notions of the soul. Matter which thinks is irreducibly matter that exists in extension, but does the adoption of a materialist perspective on consciousness deny the value of the mind–body dichotomy as an heuristic device? The ability of the body to produce meaning surely creates a distinction between thought and the more 'bovine' aspects of physiological existence, even if thought is ultimately inseparable from the body. It may not be possible to distinguish between mind and body in concrete material terms, but as a means of understanding subjectivity it is surely essential.

Even among supporters of the embodiment perspective, dualism re-emerges at the level of methodology. Neurologists have linked some thought processes with activity in different parts of the brain and different patterns of neuro-endocrinological activity. Similarly, observation of human behaviour can generate interesting insights into the human condition. However, even the corporeal topic of embodiment can only be fully grasped by adopting methods which allow the researcher to 'listen to the voices emanating from bodies'.[19] And when we listen to voices we are not primarily concerned with the vibrations of the larynx or the firing of neurons, but with accessing the meanings and interpretations produced by the informant – we are accessing a mind, not a body. So have we really transcended dualism?

Well, yes and no. Certainly the embodied perspective dispenses with the Cartesian notion of mind and body as two separate and distinct types of substance and in so doing overcomes the problem of how our thoughts are capable of acting upon other bodily systems and in turn how those other bodily systems are capable of acting on our thoughts. However, this does not represent a departure from the duality of mind and body, as Simon Williams has suggested:

> There are all sorts of ways, e.g. pain and illness, in which we experience a duality of mind/body or make analytical sense of issues in these terms. This however is at the reflective level, often in the context of a problem of some sort (cf. Heidegger's hammer) which disrupts our pre-reflective (in Merleau-Ponty's terms) or taken for granted relations to the world and our embodied being within it. I would add here, that mind emerges from body, whilst being irreducible to it . . . Irreducibility and emergence, in other words, help us move beyond either/or debates in profitable ways.[20]

Mind is not reducible to the body because it is also constituted by social experience. It is the dialectical interplay between the physiological structures of the brain and events in the external world that gives rise to consciousness. Thus, the mind is of the body yet distinct from it. In this sense the embodiment perspective does not answer the Cartesian mind–body problem, so much as reformulate the original question. Descartes' problem of how substance which thinks can influence substance in extension is replaced by an equally intractable dilemma concerning the extent to which an apparently autonomous mind is in essence bound by unconscious changes in the body, and the extent to which the physiology of the body is shaped by consciousness.

These questions of the interactions between mind–body, conscious–unconscious, internal life–social experience are ultimately empirical questions which cannot be fully resolved in abstraction. For instance, with regard to work stress we need to examine how thoughts and feelings about work manifest themselves as physiological changes, such as the endocrinological changes that accompany the stress response; how these physiological responses become embedded in the body over the life course, so that they become autonomous or unconsciously activated; the extent to which such unconsciously activated physiological responses impact on consciousness, influencing appraisals and interpretations; how both physiological responses and subjective interpretations are shaped by the outside world; and how events in the outside world are shaped by the practical activity of bodies.

Although these questions are largely empirical they do rest upon a reconceptualization of the relationships between the body, the self and the external world. These relationships can be conceptualized geometrically; for instance, Frank suggests an equilateral triangle comprising institutions, discourses and corporeality.[21] Discourses are the socially constructed 'mappings' of the body which shape our understandings of the body's possibilities and limitations; institutions are the places in which discourses operate; and corporeality refers to the physical reality of the body. The strength of Frank's approach is that it captures the way in which the self and emotional life are shaped by interactive relationships between social and physiological influences without giving explanatory primacy either to a biological substrate or to social construction.[22-3] Frank's model also demonstrates the way in which the body or body techniques mediate the interactive relationship between the individual and society; the body is viewed as both the medium and the outcome of body techniques and society as the medium and outcome of the sum of such techniques. But are Frank's triangular model and the four types of 'body use in action' he derives from it able to grasp the complex interactions that constitute the richness of embodied life?

To begin with, the three points of Frank's triangle may not address all the influences on embodied life. What about the way in which the natural world influences the emotions, body techniques and the formation of the self, and is in turn transformed into the built environment and social institutions? Secondly, the model is static, failing to account for the ways in which the self is constituted by the interplay of the environmental, discursive and corporeal across (and before) the life course, or to explain how social experiences become embedded in the body. Finally, Frank does not explore the conscious–unconscious dimensions of the self and their impact on body techniques.

The triple helix self

In place of Frank's metaphor of an equilateral triangle we would propose conceptualizing the self in terms of a triple helix. The three strands of the helix represent the external environment (the natural world, the built environment and institutions), discourse and corporeality.

Mind or subjectivity emerges from the helix as the three points spiral around each other across the life course. As well as illustrating the formation of the self at a particular point in time (the head of the helix), the model also reveals the biographical–historical dimensions of the self (the tail of the helix), as historically specific environmental conditions and discursive formations interact with corporeality across time. It is important to recognize that the tail of the helix predates the birth of the individual because corporeality (in the form of genetic material), and obviously discourse and the external environment, already exist (and already interact) before the emergence of the individual self. In this sense evolutionary pressures and genetic influences can be incorporated into the theory of the self, not as fixed ahistorical determinants of behaviour, but as dynamic aspects of the interaction between biology and the external world that emerge and are transformed over time. As well as mapping the personal biography of the self the tail of the helix also locates the individual historically, thus the external environment and discursive points of the helix describe the world at particular points in time. Thus, it is not environment and discourse in abstraction that contribute to the formation of the self, but real institutional arrangements, discursive formations, historical events, personal experiences that interact with corporeality in the genesis of the self at specific points in time and space.

Embedding

The temporal dimension of the triple helix model of the self allows consideration of embedding, i.e. the processes by which phenomena obtain a degree of fixity or continuity over time. Embedding occurs at an environmental, discursive and corporeal level.

As humans engage in practical activity (transforming the natural world, creating the built environment, making tools and producing other goods), they are embedding humanized phenomena in the environment. Obviously, there are variations in the intensity and duration of these environmentally embedded phenomena; some human activities make very little impact on the environment and what mark they do leave may be quite short-lived. Other activities, such as the construction of an urban environment, or transport systems, have a much greater and longer lasting impact on the environment. Environmental embedding has a direct relationship with the individual self, not just because it results from the externalization of human consciousness, but because embedded environmental phenomena contribute to the formation of the self; for instance, a human born into a modern western city may have a different sense of self to someone born into a low-technology third world village. So there is an interactive iterative relationship, between environmentally embedded phenomena and the formation of the self, that has existed over generations of human development. Moreover, environmental embedding can only be separated from corporeality and discursivity at the level of abstraction – environmental embedding is done by human bodies (using tools) to meet the needs and requirements of human bodies, and it is guided or informed by discourse.

Discursive or cultural embedding refers to the production and maintenance of social knowledge, beliefs and behavioural norms. As with environmental embedding there are variations in intensity and duration, with some beliefs held only by a small minority of people or for a brief 'fashionable' period, while others such as the now international systems for measuring time and the date are much more deeply embedded and longer lasting. Discursively embedded phenomena also have an interactive relationship with the self; for example, self-identity will be different in a society where religion is the dominant belief system to one in which scientific knowledge dominates. Discursively embodied phenomena also comprise 'technologies of the self'[24] i.e. belief systems employed in the reflexive management of self-identity,[25] for example, psychoanalysis, biomedicine, and narratives concerned with class, gender and ethnicity. Again there is also a corporeal dimension as discursively embedded beliefs also include body techniques,[26] such as walking, swimming, or riding a bicycle.

Finally, phenomena may also be written on the body and have a corporeal reality that is literally embedded in the flesh. The corporeal embeddedness of social experiences varies in both intensity and duration. At one end of the spectrum the faintest perception must have a physiological reality even if it is fleeting and functionally insignificant. At the other extreme, severe physiological trauma, such as loss of a limb or organ failure, are by definition deeply embedded in the flesh, and, notwithstanding the benefits of modern health technology in 'repairing' the damage and reducing the functional significance of impairment, are likely to have consequences which may span what remains of the life course, despite the individual's best efforts consciously to 'disembed' them. It is not just overt physical injuries that become embedded, but also psycho-social experiences. Over the life course social experiences become 'written' on the body in the form of physiological responses (e.g. as patterns of neurohormonal activity), some of which may also be experienced as emotional modes of feeling.[27] For instance, experience teaches us that exposure to certain external stimuli may have adverse consequences (either a physical threat to the body or an emotional threat to the self). Over time these perceptions become embedded in the body, producing the physiological and expressive correlates of fear or anxiety whenever similar stimuli are encountered.

A consequence of the adoption of a non-dualist ontology is recognition that corporeal embedding not only affects unconscious flesh, but may also affect and be affected by the mind that emerges from that flesh. Thus, psycho-social phenomena (including work stress) and their impact on mental life occur at different points on this continuum of corporeal embeddedness. In the previous chapter we questioned the trait–state dichotomy which has led some psychologists to draw a qualitative distinction between personality traits, which are claimed to be stable over long periods of time, and relatively short-term affective states produced in reaction to a particular event. We would argue that this is a false dichotomy. Rather than a bipolar opposition between fixed personality traits and short-term affective states, we would suggest a continuum of embodied emotional states that vary in terms of their intensity and embeddedness.

Disembedding

Over time embedded phenomena may be eroded by forces which are independent of conscious human activity. Environmentally embedded phenomena such as disused buildings and redundant coal mines slowly crumble away and lose their distinctively humanized form. Discursively embedded phenomena such as minority languages and traditional belief systems can also be eroded not necessarily because anyone consciously wills them to disappear, but simply as a consequence of demographic change or population migration. Similarly, corporeally embedded phenomena, such as physical injuries and affective states, may also be eroded over time through the unconscious operation of corporeal repair systems like the clotting of the blood and the homeostatic physiological mechanisms of the body.

Disembedding differs from erosion because it entails *consciously willed* effort to bring about change in environmentally, discursively, or corporeally embedded phenomena. Thus, the built environment does not just decay over time through human neglect; it is consciously transformed and reconstructed by human practical activity, through processes such as industrialization and deindustrialization. At the discursive level, belief systems are not just eroded, but consciously challenged; for example, Creationist beliefs have been marginalized by Darwinism (although the direction of discursive transformations is not always away from superstition towards science and rationality). Similarly, at the corporeal level, emotional states or modes of feeling, such as fear, anxiety, depression, humiliation, shame and grief, are consciously grappled with as we struggle to disembed them.

The adoption of a non-dualist ontology obliges us to recognize that emotional states must have a physiological reality, and, as we noted in the previous chapter, there is compelling physiological evidence to support this. There are clearly instances where individuals appear to grapple with aspects of the self that they want to change but have difficulty in changing, for example in the case of addictions, where the conscious mind might struggle to control the behaviour of a disobedient body. Similarly, individuals may grapple with other embodied experiences, such as sexual orientation, a 'bad temper', or the 'emotional scars' of a traumatic event. The key question is whether or not these physiologically embodied states can become so deeply embedded that their functional significance cannot be overcome by conscious reflection, i.e. that they cannot be disembedded by the reflexive reconstruction of the self. This question is central to the work stress phenomenon, where adverse experiences at work are frequently claimed to have left 'emotional scars' and long-term mental illness and debility. As we shall see in the concluding chapter, such claims may be 'true' for the victims of work stress, some of whom do become permanently disabled by work stress, to the point where they become incapable of remaining in paid employment; but is their fate an inevitable consequence of their experiences at work? Again, this may be an empirical question that can only be answered in the context of individual biography, depending, for instance, on the magnitude of the external stimulus or life event and the type and degree of physiological embedding. However, it can also be argued that this process is fundamentally mediated by subjective factors, i.e. the processes by which we ascribe meaning to social and physiological experiences.

The ascription of meaning is a social process at both the micro and macro levels of analysis. At the micro level, meaning is created through direct inter-action with others. In the second half of this chapter we examine the way in which the meaning ascribed to experiences at work is socially negotiated in the specific context of general medical practice. At the macro level our inter-pretations and definitions of the situation are shaped by discourse. Moreover, our beliefs about the possibility of disembedding embodied emotional states may also be influenced by discourse. In the next chapter we examine the growing tendency to make generalized claims about the fixity of emotional states arising from 'traumatic' psycho-social experiences, and the diminished sense of the self's capacity to transcend or disembed them (at least without the aid of psychotherapy).

A prerequisite of disembedding is that a phenomenon can be brought into consciousness, i.e., tautologically, in order consciously to transcend a phenomenon it must first be brought fully into consciousness. It is, therefore, essential to consider the role of the unconscious self in mediating the work stress phenomenon.

The unconscious self

The unconscious is pertinent to each of the three components of the triple helix self. At the most mundane level there may be environmental, discursive and corporeal phenomena that affect the self, but of which we are consciously unaware. Environmental factors such as early childhood poverty may affect adult health (and therefore self-identity), even though the individual concerned is not conscious of having had a deprived child-hood, or that poverty can affect health. Discursive phenomena such as modern teaching methods may affect educational attainment (and there-fore self-identity) without the individual being aware that such techniques were employed in his or her education. Similarly, the physiological processes of the body may affect an individual's mode of feeling (and therefore self-identity) without the individual being aware that such feelings have a biological dimension; for example, hormonal cycles and diurnal patterns of arousal may affect mood.

Beyond the mundane sense of the unconscious, there is a more important meaning which refers to the misrecognition or taken-for-grantedness of phenomena. Humans are born into a social world that already exists and, therefore, phenomena which are historically and culturally specific may be perceived to be universal laws of nature. Marx identified this tendency in his account of commodity fetishism:

> Man's reflections on the forms of social life, and consequently, also, his scientific analysis of those forms, take a course directly opposite to that of their actual historical development. He begins, post festum, with the results of the process of development ready to hand before him. The characters that stamp products as commodities, and whose establishment is a necessary preliminary to the circulation of commodities, have already acquired the stability of natural, self-understood forms of social life, before man seeks to decipher, not their historical character, for in his eyes they are immutable, but their meaning.[28]

Marx is not suggesting that the appearance or 'phenomenal form' of commodity production is false – under capitalism relations between people *really are* relations between things exchanged in the market – but that it presents itself to experience in a way which hides or mystifies its exploitative and historically specific essence. The phenomenal form of the work stress epidemic, i.e. which presents itself to consciousness as mental and physical illness caused by work, is equally mystifying because it hides the historical and cultural factors that have led adverse experiences at work to be interpreted through the individualized idiom of medical discourse. These historical and cultural factors will be explored in the next chapter.

Both types of unconsciousness described above affect the way in which work stress is experienced at the corporeal level, i.e. as physiological 'symptoms'. In the first sense, individuals may be aware of the relationship between particular experiences (such as adverse work characteristics) and the physiological correlates of the stress response. However, the mechanism itself is not firmly under conscious control.[29] Thus, we experience the fight or flight response as an emotional state that has swept over us, rather than as something which we have consciously willed to happen. Moreover, while we may be only too aware of some of the symptoms (palpitations, breathlessness, sweating etc.), there are other embodied responses which operate beneath the surface of consciousness.[30] Freund describes this as 'the unconsciously knowing body'.[31]

In the second mystificatory sense we are also unconscious of the way in which the pathway from external stimuli and the physiological changes of the stress response becomes embedded in the body over the life course.

How does the body unconsciously 'know' how to respond to particular work characteristics? It might be argued that evolutionary pressures have enabled the body to respond autonomically to overtly life-threatening stimuli. But most of the stimuli associated with work stress are not life-threatening. It seems unlikely that evolution would have furnished us with the capacity to respond autonomically to such recent psycho-social phenomena as low job control or lack of reciprocity in effort invested in work and the available rewards. If the bodily response to such stressors is not innate it must become embedded through social interaction and interpretation even if this process is not fully conscious. Work stress can, therefore, present itself to experience as a purely physiological response to objective conditions, effectively masking the social influences on this mode of feeling. In this sense, the stress response is self-mystifying. However, this does not mean that, once embedded in the body, the stress response becomes fixed or unvariable: 'The "schemata" or "categories" by which we "unconsciously" make sense of feeling are not static entities that simply reside in the mind. These modes of experiencing feeling originate in the body's encounter with the world.'[32]

We have suggested that the self emerges as the three points of the triple helix spiral around each other across the broad curve of the life course, during which experiences of the external world become embedded in the body. However, the observation that this process also has an unconscious dimension raises important questions about the role of conscious reflection and purposive action or social agency in the formation of self-identity. Is self-identity exclusively constituted by discourse and corporeal forces of which we are largely unconscious? If so, what remains of free will and self-determination? How do we explain how and why people consciously struggle against oppressive social arrangements and belief systems, or, at the corporeal level, how and why people struggle to exercise self-control over their bodies?

From a Cartesian perspective these questions could easily be answered by reference to the transcendental nature of the soul, or to essential and universal human attributes. However, such beliefs about human nature and the subject it gives rise to have been roundly criticized on the grounds that they claim universality for attributes which are historically and culturally specific. Michèle Barrett has summarized the anti-humanist critique of the Cartesian subject:

> Let us imagine the celebrated 'Cartesian subject'. He is made in the image of his inventor. He is white, a European; he is highly educated, he thinks and is sensitive, he can probably think in Latin and Greek; he lived a bit too soon to be a bourgeois, but he has class confidence; he has a general confidence in his existence and power; he is not a woman, not black, not a migrant, not marginal; he is heterosexual and a father.[33]

In short, humanism has falsely claimed universality for attributes and ways of thinking which are historically and culturally specific to western, middle-class men, in order to exercise power over marginalized groups by invalidating alternative subjectivities.

This critique of humanism can be traced back at least to the French structuralist Louis Althusser[34-5] who rejected essentialist theories of the self in favour of the socially constructed subject, constituted or 'interpellated' by ideology. Interpellation is the process by which ideology transforms the individual into a subject. Althusser offers two metaphors to explain the process. First, he suggests that ideology holds up a mirror in which the individual recognizes him/herself; it says, 'This is you, this what you think, what you believe and how you act.' But of course the image in the mirror is socially constructed; it reflects an identity which ultimately serves ruling class interests. Althusser's second metaphor is about hailing someone in the street. If someone calls out to us and we acknowledge them, then we accept the identity by which they hail us:

> ... ideology 'acts' or 'functions' in such a way that it 'recruits' subjects amongst the individuals (it recruits them all), or 'transforms' the individuals into subjects (it transforms them all) by the very precise operation which I have called interpellation or hailing, and which can be imagined along the lines of the most commonplace everyday police (or other) hailing: 'Hey, you there!'[36]

Althusser goes on to point out the limitations of the hailing metaphor – whereas it implies a temporal process, with a before and after, in the case of ideology there can be no before and after; the interpellation process is continual, and we are always 'in' ideology. He describes the individual as the bearer (*träger*) of ideology, suggesting a passive acceptance of ideology, rather than an active process of assimilation, thus he describes ideologies as: 'perceived–accepted–suffered cultural objects and they act functionally on men via a process that escapes them'.[37]

Althusser's virulent anti-essentialism stems from his concern to refute the claims of bourgeois humanism with its tendency to assume that socially constructed and historically specific aspects of the self are in fact universal and innate characteristics; but if subjectivity is simply 'written' onto the individual by society, where does the political will to transform society come from? As Connell has suggested, the Althusserian emphasis on structural determinism excludes the role played by 'living, sweating, bleeding human beings in their own history'.[38]

The problem of human agency is not unique to Althusser, but can also be found in post-structuralist approaches to the subject, most notably in the work of Michel Foucault. Although Foucault was one of the most prominent critics of Althusserianism,[39] he too was concerned with the ways in which social knowledge, or discourse, was implicated in the exercise of power over the individual. Particularly in his later work[40] Foucault was interested in the process of 'subjectivization', i.e. the process by which discourse constituted the subject not simply through the imposition of external constraints but through the adoption of 'technologies of the self' such as beliefs about sexuality which determine the way in which individuals construct their self-identity.[41-2] Foucault's account of the way in which the self is constituted by discourse avoids many of the difficulties associated with Althusser's account of ideology although his anti-essentialism (shared by Althusser) leads to an equally pessimistic assessment of human agency, as Giddens has pointed out:

> Foucault's history tends to have no active subjects at all. It is history with the agency removed. The individuals who appear in Foucault's analyses seem impotent to determine their own destinies. Moreover, that reflexive appropriation of history basic to history in modern culture does not appear at the level of the agents themselves. The historian is a reflective being, aware of the influence of the writing of history upon the determination of the present. But this quality of self-understanding is seemingly not extended to historical agents themselves.[43]

Much of the debate on human agency oscillates between essentialist notions of a pre-social self and the apparently agency-robbing notions expounded by Althusser or Foucault which view consciousness as exclusively the product of socially constructed discourse or ideology. Neither approach is satisfactory, but as Michèle Barrett has noted, we are not obliged to accept either:

> One does not need, having seen the errors of an overly universalistic and essentialist view of human nature, to say that there is 'thus' nothing recognisable or distinct about humans – this should be a matter for further investigation.[44]

One route out of the impasse is to define what is distinct about humans, not in terms of pre-social attributes, but as the capacity to, and necessity of, creating meaning in order to act in the world. From this perspective there is no pre-social self, indeed consciousness results from the dialectical interplay of the individual and the objective world; consciousness is always consciousness of something, and that something is the objective world.

This is the approach taken by Sartre, who describes consciousness through the metaphor of a torch beam illuminating different points in a darkened attic.[45] The contents of the attic are our memories and perceptions of the world; the sum of our biographical and physiological experiences. Sartre refers to this as being 'in itself' (*l'être en-soi*). My self-identity, i.e. who I am, what I believe, is contained in the *en-soi*. The other aspect of being (the torch beam) is simply our capacity for reflection, which Sartre refers to as being for itself (*l'être pour soi*). The *en-soi* is the raw material of consciousness; the *pour-soi* is active reflection upon it. The human mind is simultaneously being in itself and being for itself.

It is important to note that these two categories are inseparable aspects of being; there is no pre-social *pour-soi* waiting to appropriate the world, and the concrete world only exists as a set of meanings to the extent that it is the object of conscious reflection. Crucially the *pour-soi* can never be an object of reflection in itself; it is always experienced as 'nothingness', as an awareness that has no ideational content. Our consciousness of it is always as a negation of the *en-soi*, i.e. as 'I am not that'. The unbridgeable duality of consciousness, the fact that it is simultaneously *en-soi* and *pour-soi*, creates a tension: I am aware of myself as an *en-soi*, i.e. as the sum of my experiences, knowledge and biographical data, but this very act of reflection suggests to me that I am something more than my self-identity. Thus, we experience our self-identity as something incomplete, as a project to be worked on.

In attempting to achieve that sense of completeness, that unattainable unity between *en soi* and *pour soi*, we are driven to act in the world (and on the body), to experience it, produce knowledge of it, and bring it under our control. Thus without resorting to essentialist theories of a pre-social self it is possible to deduce a distinctly human mode of being, which disposes us to act in and on the world (of which the body is part); this mode of being is not characterized by a set of pre-social attributes, but by 'nothingness'.

As the torch beam in the darkened attic metaphor suggests, not all the contents of the *en-soi* can be reflected on at once. Memories, sensations, feelings drift in and out of consciousness. This process is often unwilled, for instance when sensory data push their way into our consciousness, but we also have the capacity to direct the torch beam, i.e. to call things into our consciousness, for instance when we try to remember something, or to 'make sense' of an experience, or to push unpleasant thoughts 'to the back of the mind'. This capacity for reflexivity plays an essential role in the formation and maintenance of the self – by reflecting on the contents of the *en-soi* we constantly remake ourselves in response to our experiences in the external world. In this sense the self is an ongoing reflexive project and self-identity a revisable narrative.[46]

Sartre's approach to consciousness emphasizes the extent to which we create ourselves through the choices we make as we act in the world. The centrality Sartre accords to the rational self means that his approach is richly humanist while avoiding essentialist notions of a pre-social self. However, as the triple helix model suggests, our capacity to constitute our own self-identity reflexively is limited by the corporeal reality of the body; discursive formations, including social norms, values, behavioural codes and conventions; and our relations with the external world, including the reactions of other people and our location in social hierarchies.

At the corporeal level, in order to control the processes of the body we must be able to bring them into consciousness. However, bringing a bodily process into consciousness is not always sufficient to bring it under conscious control; for example, breathing is usually controlled autonomically and most of the time it simply continues without the need for conscious reflection, although it is possible not only to make breathing an object of conscious reflection, but also to exercise a degree of conscious control over the process – either holding our breath or breathing deeply. However, there are physiological limits to this control (try holding your breath indefinitely and see what happens!). In these circumstances conscious control over bodily processes can only be achieved indirectly, by acting on the external world in a way that brings about the desired effect on the body; for example, in order to stop breathing indefinitely we need to find an external means of doing violence to the body. We will argue that this process of consciously struggling to control unconscious and semi-autonomous bodily processes is central to understanding the work stress phenomenon.

Similarly, at the discursive and environmental levels there are belief systems, institutional arrangements and social relations which have a profound influence on the formation of our self-identity, but of which we are either entirely unaware or which have become so deeply embedded that we take them for granted as inevitable, supra-historical phenomena which cannot be transformed by human activity. As Marx observed:

> Men make their own history, but they do not make it just as they please; they do not make it under circumstances chosen by themselves, but under circumstances directly encountered, given and transmitted from the past.[47]

Again, our need to make sense of, and act upon, a given society and environment provides the basis for a critical engagement with existing arrangements. Phenomena may present themselves to experience in a form which is systematically misleading or inadequate, but our day-to-day experience of acting in and reflecting on the world provides the potential for those phenomenal forms to be radically deconstructed and transformed through practical activity. Thus, the struggle to bring corporeal processes into consciousness and exercise control over them is mirrored by the struggle to bring environmental and discursive phenomena into consciousness in order to transform them through practical activity. Neither activity is conducted in isolation, but depends upon social interaction and collective activity; on the constantly changing relationship between the self and society.

The processes by which the relationship between social identity and self-identity is negotiated through social interaction in everyday life have been closely charted by Erving Goffman.[48–9] Adopting a 'dramaturgical' perspective on social interaction, Goffman explores the way in which the micro-relations of public order are maintained by techniques employed in the presentation of the self.[50-1] Unlike Maus's body techniques, Goffman's account of everyday activities, like walking, emphasizes the extent to which they are governed by interaction with others; for example, walking down the street is governed by shared pedestrian 'traffic rules' which give rise to conventions such as queues, files, processions and marches. Many of these rules are ritualized to such a degree that they barely require conscious regulation. Even so, the individual must be constantly scanning the reactions of others, not just to ensure that his or her own behaviour is appropriate and acceptable, but also to read the intentions and actions of others.

The intercorporeal aspects of social interaction, in which we both interpret the signs and behaviours exhibited by others and have our own behaviour interpreted by them, leads Goffman to explore the ways in which the surface of the body is consciously managed in order to communicate a particular message; for example, individuals may deploy 'body-gloss' (bodily gestures which are consciously adopted to communicate particular intentions). Similarly, 'face-work' may be used to communicate a particular emotional state. As the dramaturgical analogy suggests, the face we present varies according to the social context; rather than a direct and unconscious reflection of an inner state, body idiom is consciously manipulated to present a socially acceptable face even if this entails a discontinuity between outward appearance and inner feelings.

As well as ensuring the smooth flow of social encounters, these performances are also important to the maintenance of self-identity. This becomes apparent on occasions when the dramaturgical mask slips and we make a social gaffe or blunder and experience embarrassment.[52] Such instances are often countered with 'repair work', such as an apology, to restore any damage to the social self. Embarrassment can also come from 'bodily betrayal' when the outward appearance of the body refuses to conform to the self we want to present, for example when the outward signs of anxiety undermine our desire to appear calm and collected. Similarly, 'stigma symbols' such as a physical impairment or scar may create a tension between the virtual and actual social identity.[53]

It is not just momentary lapses in performance and physical impairments that can create a discrepancy between the self that we attempt to present and the self that others see and interpret. Our position in social hierarchies of class,[54] gender[55] and ethnicity is also embodied and enacted in social interaction, through our 'social style' (etiquette, dress, deportment, gesture, intonation, dialect), which further limits our control over the presentation of the self.

Despite this apparent awareness of the relationship between social hierarchies and self-identity, Goffman has been criticized for understating the power of social structure in determining the inner self, and for focusing on 'surface acting' rather than on deeper emotional states.[56] Although critical of Goffman, Arlie Hochschild has adopted a broadly Goffmanesque approach to 'emotion work'. Hochschild is concerned with the relationship between socially prescribed 'feeling rules' and the inner emotional life of the individual.[57-8] There are two key strategies for dealing with disparities between our inner emotions and what is socially expected of us. 'Surface acting' simply entails displaying the signs of emotional states that we do not actually feel, for example smiling at people we loathe. However, it is the second form of emotion work, 'deep acting', with which Hochschild is primarily concerned. Deep acting entails more than simply feigning emotion; it entails consciously restructuring what we feel, for example transforming anger into sympathy. In her study of flight attendants, Hochschild found that the demand to constantly present a smiling, helpful and sympathetic approach to passengers led to dramaturgical stress. Some responded to this with surface acting; however, behaving in such an 'inauthentic' fashion could damage self-esteem, so many resorted to deep acting, for example thinking up excuses for the rude or aggressive behaviour of passengers, in order to feel sympathy rather than anger towards them.

A key aspect of Hochschild's approach is that it links emotion work to the wage–labour nexus, describing the way in which human feelings have become commodities to be bought and sold: 'When the manager gives the company his enthusiastic faith, when the airline stewardess gives her passengers her psyched-up but quasi-genuine reassuring warmth, what is sold as an aspect of labour power is deep acting.'[59]

Critics have suggested that emotion work is not purely a product of late capitalism.[60] However, Hochschild's analysis (though more broadly applicable) is particularly pertinent to managerial structures of control in the contemporary workplace. Those who occupy positions of power and status within social hierarchies are better able to insulate themselves from 'unpleasant' modes of feeling than are the relatively powerless or low-status. Hochschild has suggested that the resources available to the powerful enable them to use 'status shields' to protect the boundaries of the self and maintain a positive self-identity. Those in relatively powerless positions, by contrast, may find their emotions manipulated as a means of social control, for instance finding their emotional responses 'invalidated' by more powerful actors, and being *obliged* to engage in 'deep acting'.

A further strength of Hochschild's approach is that it takes an embodied approach to emotional states, acknowledging that what is being reconfigured by deep acting is not simply an abstract frame of mind, but physiologically embedded modes of feeling. The fact that modes of feeling are also constructed from social experiences means that Hochschild's account of emotion work provides 'conceptual connecting tissue' between physiological and sociological models of emotion.[61]

The strength of Hochschild's approach (after Goffman) is that it returns the conscious self to the centre of the relationship between work characteristics and the body. Hochschild recognizes that powerlessness at work exposes the individual to adverse experiences which can have a physiologically embodied reality. However, this process is mediated by a conscious mode of feeling and the worker's strategies of emotion management. In this sense conscious practical activity can restructure our inner emotional life; however, although emotion work may disembed work stress from consciousness, is it sufficient to disembed the unconscious physiological manifestations of the stress response? As Freund puts it: 'How "deep" can the social construction of feelings go? While one may not consciously experience psychophysical responses to invalidation, for instance, can emotion work eliminate the responses of an unconsciously knowing body?'[62]

Lynch has found that people with high blood pressure exhibit strong neuro-hormonal reactivity when exposed to stressors, but that they do not experience this subjectively, and maintain a calm exterior. This disparity between the unconscious physiological manifestation of stress and what is subjectively experienced and displayed has been described as 'schizokinesis'.[63-4] Whether it is possible to have health-damaging physiological responses to stress, but remain blissfully unaware of stress at a subjective level, is a matter for further research. However, it is worth considering the schizokinesis hypothesis from a temporal perspective.

The point of departure for conceptualizing schizokinesis is the moment in time when physiological responses to adverse experiences or life events are firmly embedded in the body. Emotion work is conceptualized as *starting* after the embedding process has taken place, as a means of breaking the link between the physiology of the stress response and its representation in subjective experience. However, if we start from an earlier point in time before the relationship between external stimuli and patterns of physiological response have been firmly embedded, then there is clearly much greater scope for a subjective reordering of those relationships. Put simply, we must at some stage in our development *consciously* learn that factors such as low control, invalidation, etc. pose a threat to the self, in order for the stimulus–physiological response mechanism to become embedded in the body, even if that relationship later comes to operate autonomically or unconsciously. Emotion work (and other cognitive strategies) are not just about *unlearning* emotional responses after they become physiologically embedded, they are also about *learning* appropriate emotional responses in the first place, i.e. before they become deeply embedded in the body's unconscious processes. The conclusion is that while deeply embedded physiological stress responses might possibly remain even after emotion work has banished them from consciousness (schizokinesis), the process by which those responses become embedded in the body in the first place is open to conscious restructuring.

Although Hochschild's account of emotion work posits an active embodied subject responding to historically and culturally specific discursive and environmental formations, the realm of action is exclusively limited to a reconfiguration of the inner self and control over the surface of the body.

Little attention is paid to the possibility of acting upon and transforming the structural and discursive factors that give rise to the work stress phenomenon.

In the first half of this chapter we have attempted to demonstrate that although work stress can be a physiologically embodied phenomenon, which can operate unconsciously, it is fundamentally about the way in which we subjectively interpret and give meaning to social and physiological experiences and the mode of feeling that these interpretations give rise to. The unconscious aspects of our cognitive and emotional life and of many of the discursive and environmental factors that shape it mean that our experiences of the work stress phenomenon cannot be easily or absolutely subordinated to conscious rational control. However, our capacity for reflection and purposive action means that we are able to grapple with our own mental life or mode of feeling (even those aspects which are largely unconscious/ autonomous) and negotiate our relationship with the external world (again, even with those aspects that lie beyond our direct control).

It is one thing to arrive at these conclusions by theoretical analysis, but how do they fit with evidence from the real world? If work stress is really about how people make sense of their experiences at work, how they invest them with meaning and socially negotiate a mode of feeling, then these processes should be accessible to research. To address this we present evidence from a case study which looks at the way in which experiences of work stress are negotiated within the micro-relations of a particular workplace and how this process fits with the claims of other models of work stress. General medical practice, with its acute emotional demands and complex network of power and status hierarchies (both within the organization and in relationships with patients), provides fertile ground for exploration of the issues raised above.

Work stress in the health sector

Workers in general practice (and for that matter within the health sector as a whole) have not proved immune to the work stress 'epidemic'. The extent of the problem is illustrated by calls to the British Medical Association's stress helpline which received more than 6000 calls in its first two years of operation.[65] Much of the empirical research has adopted a quantitative social epidemiological perspective; for example, a recent study[66–8] examined levels of stress among employees in NHS Trusts, documenting the work factors associated with stress and the effectiveness of selected interventions. Samples of the workforce were surveyed on two separate occasions in 1994– 6 and 1996–8. The findings suggest that just over a quarter of the samples in both surveys were suffering from a significant level of stress. There were considerable differences in stress levels between occupational groups (with managers, and junior managers in particular, experiencing the highest rates, and ancillary staff the lowest). As a whole the rate of psychiatric distress cases among NHS staff was substantially higher than that recorded among British employees more generally. Larger Trusts tended to experience higher levels of stress. The work characteristics which best accounted for differences in stress levels among employees were high work demands, low influence over decisions, poor feedback on performance and high role conflict. The implication of these findings is that working in hospital Trusts has become more stressful, at least for some occupations, because of high demands, low control, and unsatisfactory managerial arrangements.

A similar story can be found in general practice, where more recent developments have threatened to undermine the continuous process of professional development that occurred during the 1960s, 1970s and 1980s, which significantly raised the status and morale of practitioners and made it an attractive career option.[69] However, evidence from several recent studies[70] indicates a lowering of job satisfaction[71] and an increase in job stress and poor mental health among general practitioners.[72] It is claimed that the major sources of stress for general practitioners are increasing demands from excessive work hours (particularly out-of-hours care), administrative burden, the emotional burden of patient care, worry about complaints from patients and conflicts of career with personal life, and increasing managerial intervention created by government-inspired changes.[73-5] Further evidence suggests that younger male GPs are at particular risk of job dissatisfaction and emotional exhaustion, and are more likely to depersonalize others.[76] Firth-Cozen,[77-8] in her longitudinal study of a cohort of medical students, followed up in 1993–94, found that 33 per cent of those who went on to become GPs exhibited significant symptoms of stress, while Appleton *et al.*,[79] in a study of 406 general practice principals, found 52 per cent to be suffering from psychiatric distress. In summary, according to this argument general practice has become a difficult place to work because of increasing demands and threats to autonomy.

Medical practice entails the infringement of powerful social taboos, for example regarding access to the body; the disclosure and discussion of intimate personal information (both about the body and the social milieu); and exposure to death and the dying. There are also potentially antagonistic relationships to be negotiated, for instance between health care worker and patient, doctor and nurse, senior partner and practice manager. All this is set against a backdrop of heavy workload and financial constraints. These factors combine to make general practice a crucible for 'emotion work', as different groups and individuals continually renegotiate working relationships and attempt to present themselves to the world as caring and competent professionals. The question is, how does this emotion work affect their mode of feeling, and does it have consequences for their subjective experience of work stress?

The study reported here sought to examine the way in which work in general practice is subjectively interpreted and invested with meaning by a range of different occupational groups, including general practitioners, practice managers, administrative and reception staff, practice and district nurses, and health visitors. A more detailed account of the methodology employed in the study is given in the Appendix; however, a two-stage research design was adopted, comprising a postal survey of 81 randomly selected general medical practices, followed by in-depth qualitative interviews with staff from the occupational groups listed above at 10 of the practices that had taken part in the initial survey. Findings from the quantitative component of the study have been reported elsewhere;[80-1] here we are concerned with the themes that emerged from the follow-up interviews.

Work stress as high job demands

As we reported in the previous chapter, a key component of epidemiological accounts of work stress is the extent to which workers are exposed to high job demands such as the pressure and intensity of work. Thus, for Karasek and Theorell,[82] a worker with a heavy workload compounded by time constraints would be classified as having high job demands which, when combined with low levels of job control or social support, are considered to be indicative of job strain. Many of the informants (from all of the occupational groups) mentioned heavy workload and time constraints as causes of stress. The following comment from a district nurse is typical:

> On the good days, I think I can do a really good job and really make a difference. On the bad days, when we are very, very busy and stressed with perhaps terminally ill patients, that can really impact on my feelings about the job because if you are really busy you feel you can't always give these patients the time that they need and that is not satisfying at all, that is quite distressing when you feel that you wanted to give more but you have got so much to do that you can't.

As the above quotation suggests, the strain associated with heavy workload is not only caused by fatigue, but by the belief that it might compromise job performance (or the capacity to present oneself to the world as a caring and competent professional), in this instance by reducing the quality of care given to patients. Many of the clinicians expressed concern that pressure of work might cause them to make mistakes in diagnosis or treatment, obviously with injurious consequences for the patient, but also for the clinician in terms of loss of self-esteem, loss of respect from colleagues, and the threat of litigation.

Although Karasek and Theorell's conception of job demands in terms of the pressure and intensity of work was highly salient to people working in general practice, the informants mentioned other job demands that were not addressed by Karasek and Theorell's model, and which may be specific to the caring professions, or at least to occupations that entail a high degree of contact with the public. The first of these additional demands was dealing with difficult patients. There were two aspects to this problem: dealing with rude/abusive patients, and dealing with inappropriate demands.

The problem of rude or abusive patients varied substantially depending on the location of the practice and the demographic characteristics of the patient list. In affluent areas the problem was mainly one of verbal abuse from irate patients, for example if they had to wait a long time for an appointment. However, for urban practices, serving a more deprived population, particularly where there was a high concentration of drug addicts and mentally ill patients, the threat of violence and physical assaults was a constant concern. This from a receptionist:

> It is upsetting, of course it is, you have people screaming at you, you know, abuse, swearing at you and abuse, nobody likes that [. . .] I have had to call the police because I thought somebody was going to attack us, we had to lock ourselves in a room once, four of us including the cleaning lady.

As the first point of contact between patient and practice, receptionists often bore the main brunt of abuse from patients, and it was frequently observed that patients could be abusive to reception staff, but then extremely polite and deferential to the doctor. However, there were also instances of doctors being attacked in their surgery, and one practice had installed 'panic buttons' and surveillance cameras as a precautionary measure. The perceived risk of assault was particularly acute for staff making home visits. District nurses and health visitors often had procedures for minimizing risk, for instance sharing information on patients who had exhibited threatening behaviour and, if necessary, accompanying each other on visits. Doctors often had similar informal strategies, particularly regarding out-of-hours home visits; one doctor regularly asked his driver (supplied by the out-of-hours cooperative) to accompany him into the patient's home, if there was a perceived threat.

Constant exposure to rude patients, and the occasional threat of physical violence, were considered by many informants to be one of the more significant demands associated with working in general practice. Although this was often perceived to be a cause of stress, many informants had developed strategies for dealing with it and for minimizing its effect on their self-esteem. It was also suggested that those who were unable to cope with such demands were likely to be selected out of general practice.

The second aspect of the problem of difficult patients related to inappropriate demands. Several of the doctors presented anecdotal evidence of grossly inappropriate demands for out-of-hours home visits, but inappropriate attendance at surgery was also viewed as a problem. There is obviously considerable scope for disagreement between doctor and patient as to whether particular symptoms are sufficiently severe to warrant a consultation. However, inappropriate demand was defined not simply in terms of insignificant symptoms. Ironically, public awareness of psycho-social models of stress and health meant that doctors were often presented with social problems that they felt lay beyond their remit, for example:

> I had somebody here today that was basically in floods of tears because she wanted me to write the letter that would get her off the assignment that she was supposed to have done for her degree. Well, you know, that is not really appropriate and I have written her a letter and it is up to the tutor whether they take it seriously or not.

The job demands arising from difficult patients, either because of their rude or abusive behaviour or their inappropriate requests for treatment, were often claimed as a source of stress, partly because they were distressing and increased the workload, but there was also a moral dimension to the problem, that often manifested itself in a distinction between 'deserving' and 'undeserving' patients. Many informants suggested that the relationship between health workers and patients had deteriorated over time. Patients were perceived to be less concerned about wasting the doctor's time, more assertive in demanding their rights, more willing to present with social or relationship problems, and more likely to resort to verbal abuse if their needs were not met promptly. There were several theories as to why these changes had occurred. Some felt that the consumerist policies of the 1980s, particularly the Patient's Charter, had raised unreasonable expectations, and that the then government's attitude towards the medical profession had eroded public support.

Another job demand experienced by people working in general practice is that of caring for people who are severely or even terminally ill, or who have severe social problems. Several informants felt that female health workers received a greater proportion of emotionally demanding work than their male colleagues, partly because community nurses (who tend to be female) have greater exposure to these stressors (because they are more intensively involved in caring for the terminally ill and because in visiting patients at home they have direct experience of social problems), but also because women are seen as more sympathetic than men. This from a woman GP:

> Women on the whole are more open to listening to people's problems. I have got a friend, a male GP who does a lot of locuming [. . .] and he hates being locum for the women. He says, he gets no medicine at all, he just gets social problems, misery, unhappiness, sadness, personal conflicts within families [. . .] Patients choose who they want to go to;

if they have got a simple problem they go and see the men, who have a simple straightforward surgery and get out at six o'clock and if they have got a complicated problem they'll wait and choose to see the women and the women have just got droves of tears in front of them all day.

Coping with emotional demands is complicated by the need to strike a balance between empathy and detachment. It was often suggested that the traditional model of professional objectivity was no longer appropriate, for instance a district nurse commented:

When I did my training thirty years ago we were always told, 'Oh don't get emotionally attached to patients', which I think perhaps in a hospital setting is okay to say but [...] in the community we are guests in people's homes, we get not only to know the patient but the carer, the relatives, the family [...] and you can't help giving something of yourself in that situation. I feel that you can't stay completely detached and give really good care and I think there is a degree of emotion that's involved there.

Although many informants felt that there was a tension between empathy and detachment, which in particular circumstances might be a cause of stress (for instance, the death of a young person, or if they felt that they had not done enough for the patient), no one reported that this was a major problem. There are several possible reasons for this. It might be that the informants were reluctant to admit to what they might have thought of as emotional weakness, or that those who were affected had declined to be interviewed. Certainly, some of the informants knew of colleagues who had been unable to cope with the emotional demands of the job, some of whom had left general practice as a result. Most of the informants, however, described mechanisms or attributes that they felt enabled them to cope with such demands. Many described formal and informal support from colleagues, i.e. mentoring and group discussions about particular patients, and sharing the care of terminal or distressing cases. Others relied on informal support from family and friends (within the bounds of medical confidentiality). Those who appeared to cope best with the emotional demands were those who had the ability to 'compartmentalize' their feelings; being able to adopt an expressive and sympathetic approach where necessary, but also able to maintain sufficient detachment to act professionally and avoid the emotional consequences of over-involvement. This ability is illustrated in the following response from a general practitioner, when asked if the emotional demands of the job distressed him:

It causes me, I am afraid to say, no emotional stress whatsoever. You do have to learn to develop, it sounds horrible I know, but you do have to develop a detached professional relationship. I mean you can be upset because they are nice people and you see them suffer; I think as a doctor if you begin to let that affect you personally then you are finished, you would then become stressed yourself, depressed and your energy would burn out and eventually you'd have to give up practising medicine. I think you can help patients far better if you remain unemotional. I don't rule out emotion, I think you have got to be warm and empathetic, you should be warm and friendly and even touch them, put your arm around them and nice warm human things like that, but when they leave the room you've got to be able to either move onto the next patient or go home . . .

The belief that the ability to maintain an appropriate degree of emotional detachment was not only good for the clinician but also for the patient was held by many informants. It seems that for occupations with a clinical role in general practice there are inevitably emotional demands, particularly regarding the tension between empathy and detachment, but that with appropriate support, and sufficient emotional resilience, these demands can be satisfactorily managed.

Work stress as low job control

A second causal factor often cited in the work stress literature is job control, which is often defined not just in terms of being able to make decisions about how the work is done (decision latitude), but also as the opportunity to use a wide range of skills in varied and interesting ways (skill discretion). A high degree of job control is claimed to offer a degree of protection against the putative dangers of high job demands. As with the job demands variable, there was evidence that low job control was salient to many of the informants, several of whom raised the issue without prompting. However, appraisals of decision latitude and skill discretion were varied and subjective. For instance, two single-handed GPs, of a similar age, with similar list sizes, and serving similar populations, made quite different assessments of the variety and interest of work in general practice:

First GP: You never know what is going to come through the door next. [. . .] there is always going to be the unexpected.

Second GP: It is a repetitious job but then a lot of jobs are repetitious; it isn't high brow intellectually [. . .] so that intellectual thing doesn't become a stimulus after a few years. I think that somehow you have got to get that mental frame, that you are in for a long haul dealing with patients, in a mundane way, day in day out through your career, and not have very high expectations that it's going to be very stimulating or challenging.

One would expect the GPs quoted above to have broadly similar experiences at work, yet their subjective assessments of the variety of their work are very different. This underlines the importance of cognitive appraisal in shaping interpretations of work characteristics and further undermines the validity of epidemiological studies which have treated self-reported data as an objective reflection of actual work characteristics.

For many informants (particularly GPs), control over their own work could not meaningfully be separated from managerial and clinical responsibilities, not least because their degree of decision latitude had consequences for colleagues and patients. In this sense, the job control variable could be extended to include control over the 'business' (particularly for single-handed GPs and senior partners); control over health care resources; control over patients' health; and control over colleagues.

Even if the job control variable is expanded to include the above factors, there was still evidence to suggest that a high degree of control could bring greater job satisfaction. This from a GP who had relinquished his senior partnership:

I used to do the finances of the old practice and [. . .] I felt that in running the business side, the financial side, as well as the other work one really had one's finger on the pulse of the practice. You knew where the money was going. You knew where it was coming from and I enjoyed it.

However, although there is a strong impetus for the GP (particularly) to take control, both managerially and clinically, the responsibility that accompanies this may be cited as a cause of anxiety or stress, and several informants who appeared to enjoy a high degree of job control also complained about the burden of management, financial worries, fear of clinical mistakes and litigation. Therefore, if a broader definition of job control is taken, which includes the clinical and managerial responsibilities described above, then the claim that greater job control inevitably leads to reduced stress[83] cannot be supported. It appears that in general practice the relationship is much more complex, and some aspects of high job control may actually contribute to feelings of stress and anxiety.

The ambiguous character of job control was handled differently by different GPs. For example, some reported opting for single-handed practice because they wanted the high degree of control that they perceived it to confer, while others chose group practice because they felt the managerial burden would be less.

Work stress as low rewards

As discussed in the previous chapter, Siegrist's[84] model proposes that work stress arises when the effort invested in job performance is not felt to be reciprocated by the accrual of adequate rewards. Rewards, in this sense, include esteem and career opportunities, as well as financial gain. In general practice there is, of course, a wide disparity in pay between the different occupational groups. Some GPs were dissatisfied with aspects of the mechanism by which they were paid, for example the tying of remuneration to post-graduate education, and others reported being 'exploited' by senior partners. However, the majority felt that the financial rewards they received were at least adequate, and, as in the following case, felt that it justified the high demands of the job:

> . . . anyone that's going to be earning what we're earning has got to be in a stressful job . . . I don't think I'd like to go out and just be standing in a car park all day taking tickets or something – the stress would be the lack of income. So from that point of view I wouldn't go out of my way to say it's stressful. It is but it's only what you'd expect to earn a good income.

It is important to note that, in the above case, the informant's stress tolerance appears to be a direct function of his assessment of the adequacy of the financial rewards of the job. Not only does this support Siegrist's model of work stress, it also indicates the subjective and social dimension of appraisal and resilience.

Other occupations in general practice are obviously less well paid, and, predictably, this was often reported as a source of dissatisfaction, if not stress. However, it was often the case that informants were prepared to tolerate low pay, because they viewed the National Health Service almost as a charitable organization; this from a practice manager:

> They can't really afford to pay us that much more than he already is so I don't want to bite the hand that feeds us. You don't want to ask for so much that he can't actually keep the surgery going.

Working for a 'good cause' appeared to influence the meaning of low pay, for some of the informants. Rather than feeling cheated of their rightful rewards, or seeing their low pay as an index of under-achievement, many informants appeared to gain self-esteem, or a degree of self-aggrandisement, precisely because there was a lack of reciprocity between their efforts and financial rewards. This perspective was particularly strong among older women managers, administrative staff and receptionists who felt that they had had their 'real career' in previous jobs outside the health sector (often before having children), and that their return to work was mainly motivated by non-financial factors. Rather than contradicting Siegrist's model, this simply underlines the importance of conceptualizing 'rewards' in more than purely financial terms.

The doctor–nurse relationship

The role of the community nurse (including health visitors, district nurses and practice nurses) is changing, with many beginning to take over some of the clinical responsibilities previously held by doctors. Some GPs welcomed this change as a way of sharing workload and responsibility. Others were more reluctant to relinquish control, either because they lacked trust in the nurses' competence, feeling that they would remain clinically responsible, or because they felt that their status and income were threatened. The GP quoted below expressed his concerns forthrightly:

> I think it's a good thing really but it isn't if they're gaining power and gaining the income that you're gaining and all that sort of thing when they're asking for enormous monies and everything. So I think if that's going to happen they can forget about it. We don't want them taking over our jobs and money and position and all the rest of it but otherwise I think it's a good thing. The idea of triaging I think that's what we're going to have to do much, much more, that the nurses are going to have to deal with the trivial stuff. But the fear is having got their boot in the door, they're very mercenary and they want more money and more position and they'll get to our position. But these highly trained GP's should be more specialist and you should get the nurses to do the ordinary mundane stuff.

Many nurses were also reluctant to see their role expanded, and felt uneasy about the boundary between the roles of doctor and nurse becoming blurred. Others were much more enthusiastic and had taken additional training to enable them to increase their responsibilities, with some becoming 'nurse practitioners'. Even here, the nurse's ability to put his or her new skills into practice depended very much upon the compliance of the GP, and this was not always forthcoming. This from a practice nurse:

> . . . he [doctor] is very territorial [. . .] After I finished my diabetic course I said to him, 'I can take over some of these diabetic patients.' I said, 'If there is a problem, you know I will get back to you about it.' He said, 'Yes, yes, yes, I will think about that.'

> *And he hasn't?*

> No, and he has come to me and said, 'I'm sorry, I will do at some stage.' I said, 'Yes, I know what you are like [. . .]' He likes to keep his finger on the pulse, shall we say. But another GP, he thinks, The less I do the better, so the nurse can do that, do this [. . .] and then you will get another one that thinks we are still the handmaiden and expects us to trot round and they know best.

In many instances the relationship between doctor and nurse was characterized by a struggle over job control, but the terms of this struggle reflected the contradictory nature of job control; in some instances doctors were eager to offload work onto nurses who were reluctant to take on additional responsibilities, but in other practices well-trained and highly motivated nurses, eager to expand their remit, were at loggerheads with their more conservative doctors. This boundary dispute over job control between doctors and nurses in general practice can be a cause of tension, anxiety, and low job satisfaction, but at least it seems to be fairly self-contained and has little effect on the rest of the organization. This is not the case with the relationship between doctor and practice manager.

The doctor–practice manager relationship

Among the practices included in the follow-up study, the role and responsibilities of the practice manager varied substantially. In some the practice manager was almost like the chief executive of a small company, freeing the doctors to concentrate on clinical matters. More often though, the practice manager was little more than a senior receptionist or administrative assistant, and the doctors did most of the management. Given their heavy clinical workload, why is it that so many doctors feel the need to be involved in management? The following quotation from a manager captures the contradiction:

> These GPs have been bleating about how stressed they are and then they want to hang on to this power [. . .] Now nobody other than a doctor they tell us can do the consulting work [. . .] Fine, get on and do the consulting work. Are you telling me that you haven't got enough to fill your week doing consulting work and therefore have got spare time to do management, which other people could do? No, they'll tell you, they've got to do it in the evenings. Well is that very sensible? There are enough skilled people around. There are people who are skilled in lobbying, in negotiating, in managing situations, organizations, money who would probably do a hell of a lot better than the GPs who are playing at it.

So why do so many GPs retain a high degree of managerial responsibility? First, there is a long history of independent contractor status, during which single-handed doctors in particular were responsible for managing their own affairs without formal managerial input. There is, therefore, a tradition of independent decision making among doctors in general practice, with the doctor's wife often providing clerical and administrative support. The growth of group practice, and particularly the introduction of fundholding, enabled the role of practice manager to develop, but, particularly in smaller practices where funding for managerial pay is limited, it is difficult to recruit well-trained and experienced managers.

Recruitment is often done informally, and the doctor's wife or the senior receptionist are often 'slotted in' to the post without going through a formal appointment procedure. At some of the practices participating in the follow-up study this had worked well, but it was often the case that the practice manager had limited managerial expertise and little credibility – still being seen as the doctor's administrative assistant rather than an autonomous manager. The following quotation from a practice manager illustrates the above points:

When I first started in general practice which was thirty odd years ago, there was no such thing as a manager. You had a doctor, invariably it was in his house; his wife answered the phone; you went in to do a bit of the admin/reception; if you were a shorthand typist you could perhaps type a few letters for him, but it has evolved, mainly over the last twenty years, or, fifteen [. . .] [the doctor] likes to handle his own finances so I don't get involved with finances. I pay some of the bills, but that's always been his baby, but that suits me, I've no argument about it. I would probably do anything, cut the flowers and give him a vase of flowers, I will do what he wants really.

Whether because of historical precedent, difficulty in recruiting sufficiently competent managers, or simply the desire to be in charge, many GPs retained a significant share of managerial work. As well as increasing the GP's workload, this could also create frustration for practice managers, several of whom felt that they were not allowed to develop or fully utilize their managerial skills. As with the doctor–nurse relationship, the doctor–practice manager relationship was often characterized by a struggle over job control, with the doctors eager to delegate some of the managerial workload, but reluctant to relinquish decision-making authority. As well as causing a degree of antagonism between doctor and manager, the scarcity of fully empowered and competent managers often meant that practices were under-managed and relied on 'muddling through' rather than on proactive strategic planning and well-structured operational management. In some instances this could undermine the cohesion of a practice, causing problems for many of the staff.

Work stress as lack of social support

As with job control, high levels of social support are thought to ameliorate the stress associated with high job demands. Again, evidence from the follow-up study revealed the salience of this variable to people working in general practice; this from a receptionist:

You know that if you need to get away then somebody will cover for you. Everybody mucks in and if someone's on holiday and so on and so forth. The majority of us are similar ages. We're mature females who all muck in together and hopefully back each other up.

Although the recipients of social support at work may benefit from it, providing such support may entail a cost to the individual in terms of increased job demands; this from a practice manager:

There's another potential big stress for practice managers, which is actually very similar to the ward sister syndrome, which is that you don't get, or you rarely get, more than about 30 seconds of concentration on any one thing because you are all things to all people. Patients want you, the partners want you, the practice nurses want you, the staff want you, people on the telephone want you because you are seen as the hub of the organization, and that is how it should be, but there is an immediate corollary to that which is that you're going to be in high demand.

Many informants wanted to receive social support at work, but not everyone was prepared to give it because it would add to their job demands. Practice meetings were an example of this; many felt that they were an essential means of communication and support, but they were often not held because of the demands they raised. So the relationship between social support at work and stress reduction is not quite as straightforward as existing epidemiological and psychological models suggest.

It was not just the provision of information or help, but the whole organizational culture of the practice that appeared to influence informants' perceptions of social support. Many mentioned the importance of a 'family atmosphere' that they associated with working in a small organization (compared to private corporations, or even NHS Trusts, the largest group practices are relatively small). When prompted, informants described this 'family atmosphere' as a kind of bond that went beyond the formal obligations of the employment contract. Some of the practices made a conscious effort to cultivate this bond, by arranging 'away days' and other social activities. This bond appeared to be well developed in smaller practices where staff turnover was low and most staff had been in post for a number of years. Some practices that had undergone 'stressful experiences' like a change of premises also claimed that their experiences had strengthened solidarity.

Where the organizational culture gave rise to a 'family atmosphere', i.e. to a cohesive social bond between staff, the relations between staff appeared to be less antagonistic and more supportive. This may be because, as was noted above, social support is experienced as a benefit to the recipient but a cost to the provider, thus where a strong bond exists between staff they may be more willing to incur the costs of providing support to their colleagues, and less likely to risk the bond by refusing support.

There was no evidence to suggest that the promotion of a 'family atmosphere' was in any sense compromised by the provision of more formal managerial devices, such as job descriptions, grievance procedures and detailed contracts. In fact, in many instances relations between staff appeared to be strengthened by clarity about expectations, responsibilities and entitlements. The key factor appeared to be that such formal mechanisms should be introduced and administered flexibly and with sensitivity. Managerial style was essential for this balance between formal and informal methods of regulating social relations at work. Where managers (and partners) were able to empathize with their staff and relate to them in ways which enhanced motivation, performance, flexibility and cohesion, there appeared to be greater job satisfaction, and possibly increased resilience in the face of high job demands.

Demonstrably valuing the contribution of colleagues was also important, particularly in the doctor–nurse and doctor–practice manager relationships, discussed above. A strong commitment to the values of patient care also enhanced job satisfaction, and not just among clinicians; for example, many receptionists were acutely sensitive to the way in which clinicians treated their patients, not just because dissatisfied patients might be abusive to them, but also because their reasons for working in general practice were at least partly altruistic and they were not happy to work in an organization that they felt had an uncaring approach to patients.

Where the above factors were present they appeared to enhance people's experiences at work considerably, and to reduce stress from interpersonal strife:

> I think if the relationship that you have with the people that you work with is fine and everything is fine then it doesn't really matter that it's a heavy workload because you get on with the people. But I think if there's a sort of personality clash within the staff then I think it doesn't matter how quiet it is at the end of the day, it's still very stressful to go into work. I think it's more important the way the people, the staff gel together and how that works.

It might be assumed that the development of an organizational culture that enhances supportive social relations at work could be explained purely in terms of the personalities of the team members, or that it simply entailed giving in to all demands. However, the practices in the follow-up study that appeared to have the most satisfactory and supportive social relations were those where the manager and/or doctors had highly developed managerial and social skills, and their approach was characterized as 'firm but fair'. Under these circumstances staff were aware of their duties and responsibilities (and their rights and entitlements), but were prepared to work flexibly and supportively, because they knew that they would be treated in the same way by their colleagues and employers. The effective combination of formal managerial procedures with social and interpersonal skills is illustrated in the following quotation from a practice manager:

> I've just [. . .] produced a grievance procedure. Most people will look at that and they will know that they'll never need to use it because the informal mechanisms within the practice are based on the principle of being fair, but if push comes to shove and they felt aggrieved [. . .] [the practice] will listen [. . .] and have to respond. So I think [one should] introduce those things in a humanistic way.

The importance of creating an organizational culture that engenders supportive social relations might seem like obvious 'common sense', but there were many instances where this approach was not adopted. The following example describes a practice manager who lacked the necessary interpersonal skills:

> [She] was a very directive type of manager, very authoritarian, very immature. She [. . .] had not got the life experience to say sometimes the right thing to do is a U-turn. Sometimes the right thing to do is to just back off. Sometimes the right thing to do is to say, 'I'm sorry, I goofed', and lay yourself open to the staff saying, 'You stupid cow.' She couldn't do that. She would have hung herself before she would have done any of those things [. . .] She would spend a lot of time in and around reception and had got the sort of management style of [saying to the receptionists] 'I've told you when you pick up a phone you must say: "Good morning, [name] Surgery".' But she's saying that when the member of staff is on the phone having the conversation. You don't do that. But she couldn't understand that.

Many of the factors that engendered supportive social relations between staff were also important in developing a satisfactory relationship with patients. Single-handed GPs, particularly, spoke about the bond they developed with their patients, suggesting that it reduced unreasonable demands, aggressive behaviour and the threat of litigation. In the following quotation a single-handed GP describes the way in which interpersonal skills can be deployed to avoid a formal complaint:

> I think I have got a good antenna to know when people are going to be awkward or not happy with what I am doing [. . .] I immediately say, 'Look, have a second opinion if you're not happy', and try and defuse the situation straight away. If I think someone is a little bit disgruntled, I will say, 'I can see you are not happy. What happened; what upset you?' [. . .] If they walk out of my room crying or unhappy, which does happen, once they get home, I will pick up the phone and say, 'You left me in a very unhappy state. Look, I am really sorry, let's deal with it. What would you like me to do?' And that would defuse a possible litigation.

Many informants felt that such a bond could best be developed in a single-handed practice, or in a group practice where each doctor had an individual list of patients.

In this section evidence has been presented to assess how well three theoretical models of work stress fit the experiences of those working in general practice. The variables of job demands, job control and social support at work, as they are conceived by Karasek and Theorell, were salient to many of the informants, as was the effort–reward imbalance model of Siegrist. However, the content of the variables had to be substantially expanded to accommodate the particular work characteristics of general practice. Similarly, the relationship between job characteristics and psychiatric distress was more complicated than any of the three models of work stress predicted. This was partly because of the particular characteristics of work in general practice, but also because of the amorphous and sometimes contradictory character of the 'stress' category, and the role of consciousness in mediating the relationship between adverse experiences at work and the stress response. This points more towards the social interactionist approach to work stress. It is to the informants' perceptions of stress that the analysis now turns.

The meaning of stress

For some informants it was merely the presence of certain job characteristics, such as heavy demands, interpersonal strife, or lack of control that constituted work stress, but other informants suggested that work stress was about the inability to cope with such factors, or the physical or psychological consequences of failing to cope. There was, therefore, a degree of inconsistency about whether work stress referred to work characteristics or their effect on the individual. This is an important distinction, because it often affected informants' beliefs about whether stress was a positive or negative experience. For instance, some informants defined stress in terms of having a highly demanding and challenging job, in which case they were likely to see stress as an exciting stimulus to action, rather than as a cause of illness. Even here, though, there was often an awareness of the importance of job control, and also the claim that people have different thresholds or breaking points. This perspective on work stress is illustrated in the following quotation from a practice manager:

> Oh, it's what keeps me going. It's what gets me out of bed in the morning. I'm lucky because I have got a job which I feel in control of most of the time. I'm in control of enough of it to not feel adversely stressed. I feel positively stressed but there's a fine line there. There are days when it definitely spills into God I'm going to pull my hair out here, I can't do this anymore. But most of the time it's about the buzz. It's about the

not quite knowing what's around the corner. It's about what keeps you sharp, but people have such different thresholds and I think that's something which people need to take into account when making appointments because if you put somebody in a post where they feel they're stretched beyond their capacity, if they feel they actually haven't got the prospect of achieving this safely then that's got to be an adverse stress.

The belief that stress can be good, and that people have different thresholds of resilience, points to the subjective element in the pathway from work characteristics to ill health. The suggestion is that this 'threshold' between good and bad stress is not purely determined by objective working conditions, but by a subjective appraisal of one's ability to cope. This assessment may be influenced by factors such as job control or social support, but such factors also have a subjective element, regarding how much control or support an individual needs in order to cope. This subjective assessment of the ability to cope, or resilience, is not just shaped by the characteristics of a particular job, or the conditions that prevail in a particular practice, but by a wide range of social and cultural factors. One GP blamed the medical press:

> I think they [GPs] are a very over-complaining lot. And I made the decision some years ago to not read *Pulse*, *GP*, or *Medeconomics* [. . .] Every week [they] go on about all the hours that GPs put in, how stressed they are [. . .] They complain all the time, so I think, why read them? They make you feel unhappy, so the only magazine that I read is the *BMJ* which I enjoy!

It would be wrong to conclude that work stress is something entirely conjured up by the press. The evidence from this study suggests that adverse experiences at work can at least lower morale and make people unhappy. However, whether or not they lead to more serious psychological or physical health problems appears to depend upon a wide range of personal, social and cultural factors that determine an individual's resilience. This raises the question of whether there is anything intrinsic to work in general practice that poses a threat to mental or physical well-being. Certainly, the findings of this study suggest that work in general practice can be extremely demanding, and that in some practices changes could be introduced to engender more supportive social relations between staff and between staff and patients which might well improve morale and job satisfaction. Whether such conditions are sufficient to cause psychological or physical illness among a significant number of staff, independently of the other personal and cultural influences on resilience, is difficult to establish.

There may well be people whose experiences of working in general practice have caused them very serious problems, but they are difficult to access in studies of this kind, because they may have left general practice, be on sick leave, or refuse to participate in the study. What can be said is that of the 10 practices that participated in the qualitative part of the study (half of which had performed poorly on the job strain and mental health measures taken in the quantitative stage), none seemed to have extreme problems with work stress among their staff. This is not to suggest that they were not extremely busy, or that job satisfaction and morale could not have been improved, only that informants appeared to be coping with their work and did not expect their physical or psychological health to be impaired by their job.

The conclusion that work stress is not a major problem for most people working in general practice is reinforced by the finding that many informants saw their job as a refuge, either from stress encountered at home, or from an earlier more stressful job. This from a practice nurse who had previously worked in Accident and Emergency:

> A&E was very, very stressful, especially towards the end [. . .] When I left it about 1991, it was at the real apex of people on trolleys in Casualty for days, not hours, days. No beds, the volume of work was unbelievable [. . .] and after a while I sort of thought, I am just getting through a shift and the patients are just getting through a shift, touch wood, and I am not able to actually give them the nursing care that they deserve. And I suppose after twenty years that you do get a little bit jaundiced and I thought of practice nursing and I thought, That is a boring job but I will have a go; it will just keep me ticking over. It is going to be mostly leg ulcers but never mind.

Many informants also felt that their work had a beneficial effect on their psychological health and well-being, through social contact, and enhanced self-esteem derived from coping with a demanding job.

The findings reported above come from just one study of a particular work setting and it would, therefore, be wrong to draw broadly generalizable conclusions from them. Moreover, the design of the study was such that it was unlikely to pick up stress-related health problems which may lag several years behind exposure to adverse work experiences. However, in spite of these limitations the case study does illustrate a number of points that might also be gleaned from the discussion of the academic work stress literature presented in the first part of this chapter and in Chapter 2.

To begin with, the findings of the general practice study illustrate the extent to which work stress is the discourse of choice when it comes to making sense of adverse experiences at work. Among the litany of workplace 'stressors' reported by the informants many of the themes identified in epidemiological accounts can be recognized. The high job demands, low job control, lack of support from colleagues that comprise Karasek and Theorell's[85] job strain model can, with a few caveats, be found here, as can the lack of reciprocity which is central to Siegrist's[86] Effort–Reward Imbalance model. However, there is also evidence to support the claim that the pathway from work characteristics to distress and illness is more complicated than a crude epidemiological model of causation would imply.

The findings presented above support the conclusion that the meaning ascribed to experiences at work plays a key role in the mediation of work stress. In Chapter 2 we discussed psychological accounts of the way in which cognitive appraisal mediates the relationship between an external stimulus and the stress response,[87] and the extent to which antagonistic social relations in the workplace influence the interpretation and definition of health problems.[88] These factors also appear to be salient to the general practice workforce as predictors of distress and dissatisfaction.

This is not to suggest that work stress is 'all in the mind', only that the physiological reality of the stress response is conditioned by subjective, interpretive factors. The theoretical developments in the sociology of emotions and embodiment discussed earlier in this chapter suggest that the experience of work stress can best be conceptualized as a 'mode of being' or 'mode of feeling'[89-90] in which experiences at work are encoded and translated into behavioural and physiological responses, some of which may not be directly available to consciousness. Put simply, work stress is a function of how workers feel about their work, and these feelings have a physiological dimension (for instance, in the form of patterns of neurohormonal activity) as well as a cognitive dimension.

The construction and maintenance of a mode of feeling about work is negotiated and contested in the workplace as workers struggle to maintain and present a positive self-identity in the face of adverse conditions and intrusive others. Siegrist's Effort–Reward Imbalance model partially grasps this process by describing the role of subjective assessments of rewards (in the form of earnings, career opportunities and positive regard from others) in shaping the stress response.[91] The case study evidence presented above reveals the extent to which the balance between effort and reward is constructed and constantly renegotiated at the micro level, as workers interact with their colleagues and with patients.

The role boundary disputes between doctors and nurses and between senior partners and practice managers is illustrative of this dialectical and to some extent contradictory process. Ambivalence about the delegation of clinical and managerial responsibility reveals the contradictions in trying to achieve reciprocity between effort and rewards. On one hand heavy workload provides a strong impetus for general practitioners to delegate, but on the other hand, delegation incurs a cost not just in terms of anxiety about the competence of those to whom work is delegated but also in the loss of status, prestige, positive regard and possibly the financial rewards that may accompany maintenance of a high degree of clinical and managerial responsibility. Thus, while delegation may provide respite from heavy job demands, it may also damage the self-identity or self-esteem of the worker, adversely affecting his or her mode of feeling about work.

The key to reconciling these contradictory imperatives is to find a means of delegating workload without losing the psychological rewards of clinical and managerial responsibility. This may involve a protracted process of role bargaining with colleagues, in which the distribution of workload and the psychological rewards of responsibility are negotiated. As the evidence presented above illustrates, this negotiation can have several possible outcomes. In some instances, relationships may remain the same, with nursing staff maintaining the traditional role of 'doctor's handmaiden', and the practice manager performing the minor administrative functions traditionally done by the doctor's spouse, while the doctor retains a high proportion of the clinical and managerial workload. Where these traditional roles cannot be easily sustained, either because the doctor's workload becomes unmanageably high or because the nurse or manager contest their subordinate role, then traditional working relationships are likely to become strained or else be renegotiated.

Under these circumstances a new role has to be constructed. It is not usually possible for nurses simply to move into the existing role of junior partner, or for the administrator to be transformed into the type of chief executive found in other organizations, because such a transformation would entail disruption of the high effort–reward ratio enjoyed by the medical profession. Instead two new subjects have to be created – the nurse practitioner and the practice manager. As both of these roles are relatively new they are constantly being contested and renegotiated at the micro level of everyday interaction between individuals in the practice, as they struggle to attain what they consider to be an adequate trade-off between effort and rewards. This negotiation can in itself be a potent source of anxiety or depression.

As Franks[92] and Hochschild[93] remind us, this struggle to protect the boundaries of the self against challenges to self-esteem is influenced by structural and discursive factors, including one's position in social hierarchies of class, occupation and gender. Thus, the general practitioner's position as an independent contractor, coupled with the statutory and cultural recognition of medical credentials, confers significant power to dictate the roles of subordinate occupational groups, and to deploy 'status shields' against their demands for a more equitable distribution of effort and rewards. Moreover, occupational groups within general practice which lack the structural and discursive power of the medical profession may be vulnerable to 'invalidation' and find that their role and mode of feeling is defined largely by others.

This might partially explain why high levels of job control appear to protect against heavy job demands in Karasek and Theorell's model of job strain. Not only is a high degree of job control socially valued as an indicator of status (at least in contemporary western industrial societies), but it also provides the social space in which individuals can construct their own professional self-identity and, to a certain degree, manage the trade-off between effort and reward relatively free from direct surveillance and regulation by their superiors. Thus, for example, while community nurses may lack the structural or discursive power to contest their role decisively in relation to the general practitioner, the relatively high degree of job control they enjoy may enable them to maintain a more positive mode of feeling about their work than their position of structural and discursive subordination would suggest.

The problem of maintaining a positive self-identity and mode of feeling about work in the face of challenges from others is also relevant to the relationship between health care workers and their patients. Many informants suggested that 'difficult patients' were a cause of stress, either because of verbal and physical abuse or because of inappropriate demands for care. There are many potential explanations for why difficult patients should be considered a cause of work stress, not least the additional workload they entail and moral concerns about wasting scarce resources. However, at a more personal level, such patients also pose a threat to the professional's mode of feeling about work, by upsetting the balance of effort and reward and challenging professional self-identity. Physical or verbal abuse represents a threat to self-esteem as it negates the status and prestige usually associated with medical practice. Similarly, inappropriate demands for service, particularly when they are accompanied by a vociferous account of consumer rights (for example, when a patient demands a home visit even though the doctor considers it unnecessary), may be experienced by clinicians not only as a challenge to their authority and status, but also as a diminution of the intrinsic rewards of medical practice if affirmation from grateful patients is important to them. Again, there are structural variations in the capacity to deploy status shields against this form of invalidation, for example several informants reported difficult patients who were abusive to receptionists, but deferential and compliant towards the doctor. It is also worth considering the extent to which government policy impacts on the relationship between health care workers and patients. Several informants felt that the doctor–patient relationship had become more antagonistic because of government criticism of the profession and implementation of a consumerist ethos (as in the Patient's Charter) during the 1980s.

The management of relationships with patients (particularly those who are either 'difficult' or whose problems are very severe) entails 'emotion work', i.e. the presentation of an exterior image of calm professional competence towards the patient, even when experiencing quite opposite emotions.[94] As the findings reported above indicate, working in general practice also entails emotion work of a different kind, stemming from the demands of responding to the emotional needs of patients – termed 'emotional labour' to distinguish it from the earlier category of emotion work.[95]

Emotional labour has at least two dimensions: one is the additional workload presented by patients whose problems are to do with emotional distress caused by relationship problems or other life events. The data reported above suggest that women health care workers are more likely to encounter emotional labour of this kind than their male colleagues. This appears to be partly situational, in that problems of this kind may be more likely to present in the patient's home, where district nurses and health visitors (who are usually female) are likely to encounter them. It was also suggested that patients preferred to see women doctors about emotional problems because they considered them to be more sympathetic and helpful, although it is not clear whether this reflects unfounded gender stereotypes or a genuine variation in skills.

The second aspect of emotional labour concerns the psychological costs of emotional engagement with patients, particularly through the experience of empathy. Empathy entails taking the role of the other, or vicariously sharing the other's problems in a way which gives rise to similar feelings. This can occur inadvertently, simply as a result of witnessing patients with severe health problems, anxiety, depression or distress, or because a patient consciously demands a high degree of empathy. Since the mid-1950s general practitioners have been encouraged to adopt a more humanistic, patient-centred approach to their work.[96] To the extent that this entails a greater degree of emotional labour, it may be a prescription for higher rates of work stress.

Several strategies exist for defraying the psychological costs of emotional labour in general practice. For example, Yoels and Clair have described the way in which clinicians utilize time constraints to rebut patients' demands for emotional labour – 'You can't tell a patient that they can't have any more of your emotional life. You can say, however, "I don't have any more time".'[97] An alternative strategy involves the maintenance of 'objectivity' or 'professional distance'. This entails what Foucault[98] described as the bifurcation of the medical gaze, i.e. a separation of the physical body of the patient from his or her socio-emotional self. Baker *et al.*[99] suggest that this capacity is cultivated in medical education (at least in North America). The implication is that this process amounts to a form of emotional repression which may dehumanize the patient and store up emotional problems for the clinician, hence the encouragement to adopt a more holistic approach and tend to the patient's emotional needs.[100] However, evidence from this study suggests that whatever costs emotional detachment may have for patient care, it may be an essential strategy for the self-management of work stress caused by emotional labour in health care workers (although total emotional detachment from the patient may also be undesirable for the health worker, if a degree of emotional involvement is felt to be one of the intrinsic rewards of the job). Work in general practice, therefore, appears to entail an ongoing negotiation of emotional involvement between health worker and patient, in which the degree of attachment is reflexively managed by the worker. The management of emotional involvement also has a visceral dimension; it is a disciplining of the embodied self.

The use of such strategies to limit the adverse consequences of emotion work and emotional labour points to a much neglected concept in academic accounts of work stress, namely 'resilience'. Thus, informants described the 'threshold' between 'good' stress and 'bad' stress, suggesting that this threshold varied between individuals. Resilience is an unpopular category because it evokes essentialist notions of innate physiological characteristics, or else of a psychological reduction to personality traits. However, the evidence reported above suggests that resilience has a highly situational and socio-cultural dimension. As Eakin and MacEachen[101] have suggested, the character of social relations at work can have a fundamental impact on the resilience of workers. Our findings suggest that the adoption of an 'emotionally intelligent' managerial style can contribute significantly to the development of a supportive organizational culture, effectively soothing interpersonal strife and enhancing the maintenance of a positive mode of feeling among workers. However, the social influences on resilience extend far beyond the boundaries of the organization. Work stress exists as a discursive formation; it comprises a distinct way of conceptualizing adverse experiences at work, a social identity that can be consciously adopted, along with codes of behaviour and a particular mode of feeling.

It is not simply the case that a given set of work characteristics will automatically produce mental or physical health problems. What workers make of their situation, how they negotiate social relations at work, how they define and interpret their experiences, and their assessments of their own mental resilience, also appear to have an effect. Moreover, the extent to which mental resilience is valued (or inability to cope is stigmatized) varies historically and culturally, and may have an impact on workers' perceptions of what is expected of them.

The suggestion is that an accurate assessment of the extent to which work stress is a problem for people working in general practice cannot be made simply by examining a limited range of work characteristics and health indicators. Rather than treating the individual as a passive responder to objective circumstances, it is important to treat the subject as an embodied reflexive actor, constantly assessing and interpreting his or her circumstances, within a broader social and cultural context.[102]

The extent to which the work stress phenomenon is consciously mediated raises a fundamental question about the work stress 'epidemic' – is it simply the case that, when all other factors have been considered, work has become so intense and demanding that an increasingly large proportion of workers cannot be expected to cope with it, or is it that social and cultural expectations of human resilience have diminished to such a degree that workers are more likely to feel unable to cope? Has work become harder, or have workers become less resilient?

Closely related to this question is the issue of 'claims making'. By shifting disputes about the structure, organization and content of work into the domain of health and safety the work stress discourse provides a means of addressing grievances which might previously have been negotiated within the framework of industrial relations or political practice. Embracing the identity of 'work stress victim' effectively transforms what might otherwise be seen as the pursuit of sectional interests into a moral claim about the provision of 'healthy' working conditions. Even disputes which appear to adopt the strategies of traditional trade union activity are often underpinned by the work stress discourse.

On May Day 2001 at least 1000 general practitioners engaged in 'industrial action' (whipped up by *Doctor* magazine), with many closing their surgeries for the day (after arranging emergency cover) and going to London to petition the Health Secretary outside the Department of Health. However, as indicated by the following quotation from Dr John Chisholm, Chairman of the British Medical Association's General Practitioners' Committee, the dispute was legitimated by concern that work stress was undermining patient care and the health of doctors, rather than by reference to naked self-interest:

> I understand and share the concerns of general practitioners. Many of them are at breaking point because of their intolerable workload. It is important that the government listens to their concerns and takes urgent action to give patients the high-quality service they deserve and which doctors want to provide – a service that protects patient health and safety, and the health of family doctors too.[103]

Not everyone was duped by the BMA's spin. Writing in the *Guardian*, Polly Toynbee noted that with a 6.1 per cent per year pay increase (over three times the predicted inflation rate) guaranteed for the next four years, the introduction of cooperatives to deal with out-of-hours care, the halving of daytime home visits over the last decade and the rapid expansion in nursing support, GPs have 'never had it so good'.[104] Predictably, the *Guardian* letters page was subsequently filled with GPs' rather tentative rebuttals, the most convincing of which came from a Doctor Sullivan of Truro: 'If the job is so good, why are so many GPs retiring early, sick and fed up, while so few are prepared to join the profession?'[105] So are GPs 'really' stressed?

Evidence from our own modest study supports the observation that many GPs explain their experiences at work in terms of the work stress discourse. However, these reports can be explained in a number of ways:

1 From a *realist* perspective it might be argued that the demands of general practice are so great that they cause physical illness which GPs then report.
2 From the *claims-making* perspective it might be argued that the demands of general practice are not sufficient to cause physical illness, but that GPs are making a false claim in order to add weight to their demands for better pay and conditions.

3 From a *social constructionist* perspective it might be argued that exposure to the discourse of work stress leads GPs to interpret experiences at work as potential health problems, giving rise to subjective feelings of stress and low morale, leading to claims making and illness behaviour.

4 The *embodiment* perspective, outlined earlier in this chapter, goes one step further than the social constructionist approach, by arguing that the mode of feeling to which the work stress discourse gives rise may itself entail physiological changes which might in turn lead to disease.

The four modes of explanation have different strengths and weaknesses and are by no means mutually exclusive. The realist argument fits most closely with the epidemiological perspective on work stress and raises the same questions – what is the pathway between work characteristics and disease? Why do some people appear to thrive in jobs which others find unbearably stressful? These questions cannot easily be answered without looking at variations in the physiological and psychological attributes of the individual. However, once psychological attributes are introduced into the equation, then all of the cultural and discursive influences that comprise the social constructionist approach to work stress must also be considered as potential influences on the formation of those psychological attributes.

The claims-making perspective, on the other hand, overlooks the lived experience of work stress, and, as well as assuming a massive act of bad faith on the part of work stress 'sufferers', also fails to account for the empirical evidence that attributions of work stress really are associated with mental and physical health problems, even when no personal or collective 'claim' is being pursued, for instance in the anonymous responses to survey research. The social constructionist and embodiment perspectives overcome these difficulties by looking at the way in which social and cultural factors impact on the way people make sense of and ascribe meaning to their lived experiences in the workplace and the consequences that this process may have for their mental and physical health. However, the question still remains as to the extent to which the current 'epidemic' of work stress is primarily a function of changes in the structure, organization, intensity and content of work, or of cultural and discursive changes that have transformed the ways in which we make sense of our experiences at work and have sapped our resilience. This question is addressed in the following chapter where changes in work and resilience are considered from a macro perspective.

 **4** ## A brief history of work and emotions

Has work become harder or have workers become less resilient? This seemingly straightforward question is surprisingly difficult to answer. Many people would presumably agree that their experiences of paid employment are quite different to those of their grandparents, or even their parents, but are these changes the same for all workers? When did they occur? Are they uniformly for the worse or for the better? The experience of work is so variable, so multifaceted, and so individualized that a simple yes or no answer to the question of whether work has become harder is immediately open to refutation by evidence of the opposite tendency. The safest, if rather unsatisfactory, position is that work is better in some ways and worse in others and that the net gain or loss will vary from group to group if not from person to person. Despite the apparent need for circumspection many commentators have made generalized claims about historical changes in work; marking the transition from Fordism to post-Fordism,[1-2] the 'Brazilianization' of work in the West,[3] or the emergence of 'flexible capitalism'.[4] The consensus appears to be that things are getting worse.

If anything, generalized statements about historical changes in 'our' mental and emotional resilience are fraught with even greater difficulties, because our experiences are so subjective, variable and individualized. Examples of mental frailty spring easily to mind, not least from the field of work stress; for example, the Newport teacher Janice Howell, awarded £254,362 in compensation after suffering a nervous breakdown which she claimed was due to the 'two-year nightmare' of teaching 11 children with special educational needs in a mainstream class of 28,[5] or Gary Maddock, the former ambulance driver who sought £400,000 in compensation from his employers, because his experiences at work had left him so traumatized that he could no longer stand the smell of roasting meat.[6] However, against these accounts of mental vulnerability it is also possible to find instances of extreme resilience and endurance, for example round the world yachtsman Tony Bullimore who, after surviving four nights under the hull of his capsized yacht in the hostile seas of the Southern Ocean, famously claimed that he would prefer a pint of beer to a counselling session.[7] Yet despite these occasional acts of heroism commentators have still concluded that we live in a culture of victimhood,[8] and therapy,[9] in which expectations of human resilience have diminished and the use of psychotherapy has rapidly expanded.

The aim of this chapter is to explore the claims that have been made regarding historical changes in work and emotional resilience and the empirical evidence that supports such claims. While we might not arrive at all-encompassing conclusions we may at least identify underlying trends and tendencies. We begin with the changing face of work. The evidence presented below is largely drawn from the British context although, with a few caveats, similar changes have occurred in the USA and continental Europe.

Changes in work

When the public discourse of work stress was examined in Chapter 1, we observed that the phenomenon was premised on the belief that paid employment took a sudden turn for the worse somewhere in the mid-1970s, which substantially increased the pressures and demands placed on the worker. This claim fits in with popular perceptions of the social, economic and political history of post-war Britain, which posits a 'golden age' of increasing affluence, economic growth, extensive welfare provision, workers' rights and trade union power that extended roughly from the early 1950s through to the economic slump of the mid-1970s. It is often suggested, particularly by commentators on the right, that this golden age of employment came to an end because the pendulum had swung too far in favour of workers' interests and away from those of employers, shareholders and consumers. The trade unions were too powerful and were effectively able to 'hold the country to ransom' in the pursuit of ever more generous improvements in pay and working conditions. Nationalized industries, heavily dependent on public subsidies, had become grossly inefficient, lacking the entrepreneurial spark needed to modernize and respond to consumer demands. Employment rights and job differentiation had made the British workforce inflexible, lowering productivity and making Britain uncompetitive in an increasingly global economy. It was widely held that Britain was paying itself too much for doing too little work. The post-war settlement between labour and capital, based on Keynesian economics, full employment and extensive welfare provision, was no longer sustainable.

Matters came to a head in the mid-1970s, when the Organization of Petroleum Exporting Countries (OPEC) instigated a sharp increase in oil prices which led to global recession, and the International Monetary Fund refused to underwrite the Wilson government's public spending plans unless radical changes in economic and social policy were implemented. The IMF's insistence on neo-liberalism effectively brought the post-war social democratic agenda to a close, ushering in governments of the New Right. In Britain, Margaret Thatcher's Conservative government came to power in 1979 and quickly began dismantling employment laws that had protected the interests of workers. Trade union rights were swiftly curtailed (a theme we shall return to later in the chapter), nationalized industries were privatized, tax cuts were introduced and attempts were made to rein in public spending, through cuts in services.

These changes, implemented throughout the 1980s and early 1990s, changed the industrial and commercial landscape of Britain. Traditional manufacturing and extractive industries went into sharp decline, creating record levels of unemployment particularly in the early 1980s and again in the early 1990s. Communities that had grown up around single industries such as coal mining, steel making or ship building, where the same jobs had been passed on for generations, found that their traditional way of life was no longer tenable.

Not only did Thatcherism decisively swing the pendulum back in favour of employers and shareholders and away from the interests of workers; it also aimed to create a new moral climate. Mrs Thatcher was fond of expounding her version of 'kitchen table' economics: a combination of thrift and hard work – only spending what has been earned. It was not enough to cast off the structural and institutional constraints on the free operation of markets, but necessary to incite a new culture of entrepreneurship and innovation. Traditional expectations of a 'job for life' and the fixed routine of many jobs in the Fordist era would be replaced by a new ideology of 'flexibility' and change. The Taylorist image of the production line worker repeatedly performing a routine task over and over again, for the same company, over the course of a long and predictable career, was replaced by that of the dynamic multi-skilled team worker, taking the initiative, performing a range of different tasks as and when needed, and being prepared to retrain and change employers or even geographically relocate, as short-term employment contracts expired, and fluctuations in the market dictated change.

As well as the radical 'reforms' implemented by government the 1980s also saw the emergence of new managerial strategies, such as 'just-in-time' production, and 'total quality management' that led to much tighter surveillance and regulation of production, facilitated and enhanced by the more extensive use of information technology. All of these techniques aimed to boost productivity and profitability by intensifying the labour process – squeezing more work out of the individual worker. Corporate mergers, 'downsizing' and the 're-engineering' of traditional industries had produced leaner and more flexible companies better able to compete on global markets, but at what cost? By the mid-1990s many British workers, it is argued, faced greater job insecurity, fewer rights at work, a longer working week, and increased pressure to work harder. Had the pendulum swung back too far in favour of employers at the expense of workers?

Certainly, the political climate had changed in the twenty years between 1975 and 1995. Tabloid headlines about benefit 'scroungers', industrial disputes, 'red tape' and inefficient nationalized monopolies had been overtaken by stories about 'fat-cat bosses' receiving massive pay increases far in excess of those of their workers, the appalling state of underfunded public services and their overstretched staff, and social problems such as crime, inner city deprivation, and drug addiction that were increasingly seen as consequences of the economic changes introduced in the 'greedy', self-interested eighties. Thus, 1997 saw the election of a Labour government committed, at least rhetorically, to achieving a more equitable balance between economic and social interests, not least between employers and workers.

It is not surprising that the work stress phenomenon, which had existed in one form or another for at least forty years, should suddenly come to prominence. It fitted so well with the political climate of the time; specifically the belief that the interests of workers had been cast aside to satisfy the needs of a vigorous global capitalism. It took little imagination after twenty years of laissez-faire economics, trade union bashing, factory closures, pay cuts, record peaks in unemployment, productivity deals, privatization and belt tightening, to believe that the pendulum had swung too far in favour of the bosses and that workers were quite literally being pushed to the brink of mental and physical collapse. But is it true? The transformation of work during the 1980s may not have been in workers' best interests, but was it really sufficient to damage their health? To answer this question we need to look more closely at the changes in work described above, and to extend the analysis back beyond the 'golden age' of employment that is claimed to have occurred during the third quarter of the twentieth century. We begin by looking at job insecurity.

Job insecurity and job tenure

There is an ironic, or even paradoxical aspect to considering job insecurity as a cause of work stress because it concerns the threat of unemployment rather than intrinsic characteristics of the work: to adapt a Wildean aphorism, it seems the only thing worse than having a 'bad' job is the prospect of losing it. Moreover, it is important to distinguish between subjective fears that one's job is at risk and the objective reality of changes in job tenure. To this we must add the question of personal choice; what proportion of people change jobs frequently in pursuit of self-advancement, and what proportion are forced to move through compulsory redundancy or the termination of a fixed-term contract? Burchell *et al.*[10] make the point that job insecurity is not just about the fear of unemployment, but also the threat to valued job features, such as promotion prospects and levels of pay, that might result from organizational restructuring or from redundancy and re-employment. The balance of costs and benefits of changing jobs varies depending on particular circumstances. For instance, a young worker in a new industry (for example, information technology), whose skills are in short supply, may well be able to bargain for better pay and conditions by changing (or threatening to change) employers, but older workers, in traditional manufacturing industries which are in decline, may have much less bargaining power particularly if job change is forced, through downsizing or plant closure. Using US government data, Richard Sennett has demonstrated that today the percentage of workers who significantly lose out by moving jobs (34 per cent) outweighs the percentage of those who significantly gain (28 per cent). A generation earlier the percentages were reversed, with more workers gaining than losing.[11]

In assessing the impact that job insecurity might have on work stress it is also important to consider the intensity or specificity of the threat. For example, several plant closure studies suggest that the period between the announcement of closure and actual job losses (which can extend over many months) can cause acute mental distress among workers, greater even than that found during the subsequent period of unemployment.[12] However, the effects might be quite different where the threat of unemployment remains a possibility rather than a certainty.

To the evidence then. We begin by considering changes in job tenure, i.e. the average length of time spent in a particular job. We noted above that the demise of 'a job for life' is a common theme in both public and academic discourses on work. The globalization of production has created a situation where companies need to respond rapidly to changes in demand, as Beck has suggested:

> Depending on whether the dollar rate of exchange goes up or down, interest rates rise or fall, East Asian or South American banks and markets totter, whether Greenpeace intervenes and consumers stage an eco-revolt, whether governments raise petrol prices and lower speed limits, whether companies market new products, merge or split or suddenly vanish – according to all these factors, the order-book situation, investment decisions and management strategies change from one year to the next, from one quarter, or sometimes even one week to the next.[13]

One consequence of this uncertainty is the need for employers to exercise greater control over the size of their workforce; to be able to 'hire and fire at will', in order to respond to fluctuations in demand and to increase efficiency through corporate 'downsizing' or 're-engineering' – hence the changes in employment legislation during the early 1980s and the rise of the fixed-term contract and consultancy work. The image conjured is that of a mass of itinerant workers, drifting endlessly from one short-term job to another. But how accurate is this impression?

A study of member countries of the Organization for Economic Co-operation and Development (OECD) in 1997 found that, despite the popular perception of job insecurity, average job tenure or the likelihood of staying in a job had changed little.[14] Similarly, a recent British study[15] suggests that average job tenure has remained relatively stable since 1975. However, the average masks gender and age differences. The slight (2–5 per cent) decline in job tenure among men and women without children has been offset by improved tenure among women with children (which appears to have been bolstered by improvements in maternity leave rights). There are also significant differences between age groups. Younger workers tend to change jobs more frequently than older workers and this tendency appears to have increased over time. Thus, between 1975 and 1985 median job tenure for under-25s fell by 30 per cent from 1 year and 10 months to 1 year and 5 months, and by another 7 per cent by 1995. Average job tenure among men over 50 fell from 15 years and 3 months to 13 years and 8 months. So there does appear to have been a small decline in job tenure at least for some groups of workers, but hardly the radical transformation suggested by some commentators.

Even if there has been little change in actual job tenure since 1975 it might be argued that the subjective fear of job loss has risen sharply, perhaps causing workers to intensify their labour in order to avoid dismissal. Regrettably, the lack of time series data means that little is known about subjective perceptions of job insecurity prior to 1986. However, reliable survey data[16–17] do show that the proportion of British workers who felt that the chances of losing their job during the next year were non-existent or unlikely remained at around 80 per cent in 1986 and 1997. Again, the aggregate figure hides variations between groups. While workers in manufacturing and sales felt more secure in 1997 than they had a decade earlier, those in the professions, the financial sector and other highly paid groups felt less secure. The economist Francis Green has suggested that it is this redistribution of insecurity towards the middle classes that accounts for its high media profile:

> All the modern hype about work insecurity forgets that capitalism is a system that has always had some insecurity in it. But only when it hits the 'chattering classes' does it appear to become an issue for public discussion.[18]

Green's analysis also questions the assumption that job insecurity keeps people 'on their toes' and causes them to work harder; data for 1997 suggest that of those who felt that the chance of job loss was zero or unlikely,

73 per cent reported putting a lot of effort into their work, compared with 71 per cent of those who felt that there was an evens or worse chance of losing their job within the year.[19] This leads into the closely related question of the long-hours culture.

Length of the working week

As with job insecurity, the empirical evidence concerning the emergence of a long-hours culture in Britain does not fit easily with the public discourse of the increasingly hard-pressed worker obliged to extend the hours of the working week in response to employers' demands and job insecurity. This is particularly evident when long-term historical trends are considered.[20] In the middle of the nineteenth century London's fitters and turners worked an average of 58.5 hours per week, virtually every week of the year. However, by 1968 manual workers not only enjoyed two to three weeks paid leave per year, but their average working week had fallen by a third to 40 hours. A similar pattern is found for all workers for whom reliable data are available. But what about more recent trends, particularly since the 'watershed' period of the mid-1970s after which the 'golden age' of employment is widely alleged to have come to an end?

In fact the historical decline in the average number of hours at work per week (excluding unpaid overtime) continued to fall, from 39.2 to 35.5, and the proportion of employed persons working at least 48 hours per week fell from 18.4 per cent to 16 per cent over the same period.[21] The United Kingdom appears to be broadly in line with the rest of Europe in terms of the average length of the working week.[22]

As with the evidence concerning changes in job tenure, the historical decline in the average number of hours worked conceals a number of changes which only emerge through more detailed analysis. First, there is some evidence of a polarization in the number of hours worked, with an increase in working hours among some groups being cancelled out by a reduction among other groups.[23] Moreover, consideration of paid and unpaid overtime (rather than contracted hours) suggests that the average working week may have actually increased during the 1990s. In 1988 full-time male employees worked an average of four hours overtime per week, but this had risen to seven hours by 1998 (for women the rise was from three to six hours per week).[24] But what does this signify? Is it that employers are able to demand more of their employees because of the fear of unemployment, or are employees choosing to take on additional overtime to boost their income or (in the case of unpaid overtime) to increase their promotion prospects? There is evidence of occupational differences in paid and unpaid overtime; the 1990s saw an increase in unpaid overtime among professionals and managers, but it remains rare among other occupational groups, many of which have shown an increase in paid overtime. Average increases in unpaid overtime might reflect the changing structure of the workforce with fewer workers in traditional blue-collar jobs (where overtime payments are usually made), towards white-collar managerial and professional jobs (where additional hours at work are often unpaid). It should also be borne in mind that unpaid overtime is a much more malleable concept than is paid overtime and may be vulnerable to cultural influences on self-reported data; that is, employees might overestimate the amount of unpaid overtime they work in response to the perceived social desirability of working long hours.

Even if we accept that workers are working longer hours as a result of pressure from their employers or broader social influences rather than through personal choice, it is worth questioning whether an average increase of two or three hours per week is in itself sufficient significantly to undermine psychological and physical health, particularly when the number of hours worked remains considerably lower than that faced by earlier generations – why was there no work stress epidemic in the 1850s when most workers were putting in a 60-hour week with no holidays? If the evidence that we are working increasingly long hours is less than convincing, is it the case that we are putting in more effort and accomplishing more work per hour than in previous times?

Work intensification

The question of work intensification has been extensively researched through-out the 1980s and 1990s, but there are methodological difficulties.[25] Organizational case studies have combined ethnographic data with analysis of written agreements and productivity deals to gain an insight into changes in work effort. Such studies have tended to show that the 1980s were a period of work intensification in Britain, particularly in the manufacturing sector, and that the subsequent increase in productivity was largely attributable to greater effort rather than an increase in skill deployment.[26-7] Although such evidence is persuasive, there are questions about whether evidence from particular organizations or sectors of the economy can be grouped together in a way that allows for generalization to the economy as a whole.

A second approach is to consider quantifiable proxies of work effort, such as an increased rate of industrial injuries,[28] a rise in the rate of dismissals,[29] or an increase in productivity in the absence of investment.[30] Thus, Nichols has suggested that the rise in fatal industrial injuries during the early 1980s (following a long historical decline) is evidence of increased labour intensi-fication.[31] However, as with other proxy indicators, there is a difficulty in ensuring that the claimed relationship is not confounded by other variables, in this instance changes in health and safety at work regulations and aware-ness, and technological changes.

The techniques of scientific management have also been brought to bear on the intensification debate. Measurements of changes in work speed were collected by external assessors from a series of factories and used to produce an index of the Percentage Utilization of Labour (PUL), which appeared to provide 'objective' evidence of increasing work intensification during the early 1980s.[32] However, the PUL has been extensively criticized for overlooking the influence that workers may have on the supposedly objective appraisals of external assessors and the impact that changes in the organization of work may have on the reliability and validity of the method.[33]

In the absence of a definitive objective measure of changes in work effort, researchers have turned to the subjective appraisals made by workers. There are essentially two approaches. The first collects retrospective data asking workers to compare their current work effort with that in their past. Thus Burchell et al.,[34] in their study of 20 workplaces, found that 64 per cent of workers claimed that they had experienced an increase in the speed of work over the past five years, and 61 per cent reported an increase in the effort they put into their jobs over the same period. Other retrospective studies have yielded similar findings.[35-6]

There are obviously problems with the retrospective methodology relating to the accuracy of recall and the possibility that responses will be influenced by cultural factors, i.e. public perceptions about changes in work. To overcome these difficulties, a second approach has been adopted which asks the same questions at two separate points in time and compares responses. Francis Green[37] has adopted this approach using data from a series of British surveys. Green's analysis begins with an examination of changes in work effort between 1992 and 1997, using data from the *Employment in Britain Survey* of 1992 and the *Skills Survey* of 1997, both of which were based on large representative samples of British workers aged 20 to 60. The same two questions were included in each survey; one referred to 'discretionary effort', i.e. the effort that a worker puts into the job beyond what is required, and the other asked about 'constrained effort', i.e. the effort demanded by the job. The percentage of men claiming to invest a lot of discretionary effort in their work did not increase significantly (67.1 per cent in 1992 and 68.5 per cent in 1997), although the increase was greater among women (69.9 per cent to 75.9 per cent). The main increase in work effort came not from personal choice but from the constraints of the job. Thus, the proportion of men who strongly agreed that their job required them to work very hard rose from 30.5 per cent in 1992 to 38.2 per cent in 1997, while the comparative figures for women workers show an increase from 33 per cent to 42.1 per cent. Green concludes that the 1990s have seen a significant intensification of work. Regrettably, the two work effort questions were not included in surveys conducted in the 1980s. However, in an interesting analytical twist Green has used alternative data to shed light on work effort trends since 1986.

This is achieved by statistically demonstrating that data relating to the sources of the pressure to work hard are positively correlated with effort and can, therefore, be combined into a quantifiable proxy. Having established this relationship Green is able to use data on the sources of work pressure (collected in 1986, 1992 and 1997) to identify changes in work effort since the mid-1980s. Respondents in the three surveys used by Green were all asked the following question: 'Which, if any, of the things on this card are important in determining how hard you work in your job?' Seven options were offered: a machine or assembly line; clients or customers; supervisor or boss; fellow workers or colleagues; one's own discretion; pay incentives; reports and appraisals. Respondents could tick as many responses as they wished. Green assigned a score of one to each of the factors ticked and summed them to produce an 'Effort Pressure Index' (EPI), ranging from 0 – no factors, to 7 – maximum pressure. Mean EPIs were then calculated for each of the three data sets.

Using the data from the two work effort questions asked in 1992 and 1997 Green was able to demonstrate a positive correlation with the EPI means for those years, effectively demonstrating that EPI is a valid proxy indicator of work effort. Thus, comparison of the EPI means for each of the data sets tells, as Green suggests, 'a strong story' about the intensification of labour between 1986 and 1997. In 1986 the EPI mean for all employees was 1.92, by 1992 it had risen to 2.41, and by 1997 it stood at 2.74. The trend was steeper for women than for men.

Green's evidence of rising work effort from the mid-1980s is convincing because it avoids the problems of using retrospective appraisals. However, as we suggested in our analysis of the epidemiological models of work stress (Chapter 2), self-reported data of this kind may be just as much a product of the dominant culture as they are of objective working conditions. As well as transforming employment law, the neo-liberal governments of the 1980s promoted a moral ideal of the highly motivated, flexible, high-performing worker, often defined in contrast to the supposedly cosseted and feckless worker of the 1970s. In many respects, this moral ideal was little more than a reaffirmation of the Protestant work ethic, and 'stress' was increasingly portrayed as a 'badge of honour' denoting close adherence to the values of hard work and asceticism. Old moral imperatives fade slowly and in many instances New Right Man is still with us. However, during the 'caring' 1990s this moral ideal was increasingly challenged. Political rhetoric about reducing red tape, freeing the entrepreneurial spirit, and promoting self-interested increases in performance was slowly contested by the belief that workers' rights had been eroded, that they had been pushed too far by coercive employers. It was at this point (the early 1990s) that the 'work stress victim' emerged as a central figure in public discourse (see Chapter 1), effectively pathologizing the workplace and lowering expectations about the scope for further improvements in human performance. At the height of

1980s yuppiedom the prophetic Hollywood movie *Wall Street* provided a moral parable not just about the anti-social character of self-interest, 'greed is good,' but also about the negative personal consequences of assuming that 'lunch is for wimps'. In the 1990s this theme gained momentum, with concerns about achieving an acceptable work–life balance, and the dangers of trying to 'have it all' becoming an increasingly prominent feature of public discourse. Under these circumstances it is perhaps not surprising that workers should become increasingly aware of the effort that paid employment demands from them and that self-reports of work effort should show a steady rise from the mid-1980s onwards. This is not to suggest that the recorded intensification of work is entirely explicable in terms of the influence of discourse, independently of actual changes in work, just that the problematization of work may be a consequence of both.

Before leaving Green's work it is worth looking more closely at the components of the EPI. We have already noted that the intensification of work during the 1990s came mainly from an increase in constrained effort (what the job demands), rather than from discretionary effort (personal choice). Further light is shed on this distinction when the EPI components are examined. In 1986 personal discretion was overwhelmingly the most commonly reported determinant of how hard people worked – selected by 61.5 per cent of workers. This figure rose to 65.1 per cent in 1992 and to 67.6 per cent in 1997. However, although personal discretion remained the most common, other sources of effort increased more rapidly during this period. Thus, the second commonest source of effort in 1986 was 'clients and customers' reported by 37.2 per cent, but this had risen dramatically to 53.9 per cent in 1997. Even more dramatically, the percentage of workers citing 'fellow workers or colleagues' as a determinant of hard working rose from 28.7 per cent in 1986 to 57 per cent in 1997. The rates reporting 'pay incentives' rose from 15.3 per cent to 29.8 per cent, 'reports and appraisals' rose from 15.3 per cent to 23.5 per cent, 'supervisor or boss' from 26.7 per cent to 41 per cent, and 'machine or assembly line' from 7.1 per cent to 10.2 per cent. These figures do not fit well either with the claim that workers are being coerced into working harder against their will, or, alternatively, that they are freely choosing to work harder. Rather, they suggest a combination of 'sticks and carrots' that have made workers more conscious of the pressure to work hard. Of course, the technical term for sticks and carrots is management.

Management and flexibility

At first glance the notions of flexible working and managerial control might be assumed to stand in opposition to each other. The central components of flexibility: teamworking, flexitime, home working, zero-hour contracts, multi-skilling, multi-tasking, are all inconsistent with traditional hierarchical and bureaucratic managerial structures of control. However, as we shall see, rather than loosening the grip of management and empowering the worker, these developments have actually increased the scope of managerial domination and subordinated the worker to ever greater managerial surveillance and regulation.

Many of the developments that characterize the new management can be grouped under three innovations: 'Just In Time' (JIT) production, 'Total Quality Management' (TQM), and 'Human Resource Management' (HRM). By 1996 these new ways of working could be found in 70 per cent of British manufacturing sites.[38] And many aspects of these developments can be found in virtually all sectors of the economy, private and public. The aim of JIT is to increase efficiency and flexibility by reducing inventories and avoiding the stockpiling of goods. This is achieved by exerting greater control over workflow. More extensive use of information technology has facilitated the implementation of JIT production, and the development of contractual penalty clauses for late delivery or poor quality of goods and services has increased the need for tighter controls.

TQM entails the continuous search for quality improvements at every level of an organization. Workers are not only expected to contribute to the development of new quality initiatives, but are also bound by mechanisms of quality control. Both JIT and TQM depend upon changing the ways in which workers are organized, regulated and rewarded. This process and the techniques it entails fall under the remit of Human Resource Management. Multi-skilling is developed through job rotation or training in order to enable workers to perform a wide range of functions within an organization. Such workers can then be redeployed on different tasks to avoid idle time; for example, skilled engineers responsible for maintaining the smooth running of, say, a bottling plant can be used to pack bottles, if their technical skills are not required to repair a breakdown. Not only does muti-skilling reduce the number of employees needed (and therefore salary costs), it also maximizes labour use by avoiding slack periods when workers have little to do. Information technology (IT) further enhances control over workflow, by enabling workers to be constantly presented with an optimal supply of work. For example, in a modern telephone call centre IT is not only used to monitor the time taken in dealing with each call; it is also used to ensure that a new call is presented as soon as the last one has ended. Some commentators have described this as 'management by stress'.[39–41] However, others have found that where such measures are implemented with the involvement and consent of workers then job satisfaction can be enhanced.[42]

Theoretically there appears to be a degree of confusion over the consequences of many of the new managerial arrangements. At the height of Fordism, when factory workers were deskilled and subordinated to the discipline of the assembly line and Taylor's time and motion studies, critics from Charlie Chaplin in his film *Modern Times* through to the American

Marxist Harry Braverman[43] railed against the deadening routine and dehumanizing character of capitalist production in which the worker was little more than a cog in a machine. Indeed, many of the characteristics of flexible working, such as multi-skilling and teamworking, were proposed as a means of enriching the experience of work and reducing stress.[44] However, now that such practices are commonly found not just in manufacturing but in many other sectors of the economy, critics have recognized that they are not a panacea for the ills of the workplace; indeed, Richard Sennett has suggested that 'teamwork is the group practice of demeaning superficiality.'[45]

The problem is that many of the practices ushered in by the new managerialism are little more than a parody of traditional socialist conceptions of how work should be organized. Despite appearances, multi-skilling does not equal an assault on the division of labour, teamworking is not collective working, delegation and empowerment do not equal workers' control, and flexitime and home working do not represent the end of bossing. Beneath the democratic veneer of the new managerialism traditional capitalist production relations remain firmly in place – workers are still obliged to sell their labour power in the market, goods and services are still produced for exchange, managers continue to control the processes of work, and shareholders continue to extract a profit. In this context multi-skilling means never having a break, flexibility means job insecurity, teamworking amounts to an abnegation of responsibility by managers, and new technology is just another means of increasing the workload.

A key aspect of the new managerialism is the extent to which it represents a transformation of the exercise of managerial control. In some respects the introduction of new technology has simply extended the 'overseer' role of the factory foreman, enabling many forms of work to be constantly subjected to surveillance and regulation, even outside the formal workplace (through e-mails, laptop computers and mobile phones). However, the more significant transformation has come in the extent to which managers have attempted to instil corporate values and the managerial world view into the minds of their employees. The dissemination of corporate mission statements and objectives, the development of a corporate identity, team-building exercises (those dreaded paintball and survivalist outings on Dartmoor), incentive schemes and consultation exercises all aim to give workers a sense of commitment to corporate goals and diminish the culture of opposition and antagonism that characterized industrial relations in the past. The aim is to increase self-governance, so that workers will not just work hard for the company when they are directly observed by management, but will internalize the corporate agenda to such a degree that they will continue to pursue its objectives vigorously even when their activities are not being supervised. The payout is not just in terms of increased productivity, but in undermining the basis for collective oppositional activity. This leads into our next theme concerning the transformation of the trade unions.

The changing face of British trade unions

In February 1997 the authors commenced a pilot study examining issues of work and health among employees of a large shipping company. We had met with one of the company's local managers who had granted us permission to use personnel records as our sampling frame and to obtain names and addresses for the postal questionnaire. A small number of pilot questionnaires were despatched and we looked forward to analysing the provisional data. One of us took the opportunity for a brief holiday in the Lake District, and on his return found his answerphone filled with a series of increasingly irate messages from the company, the last of which threatened legal action against the university and the agency that had funded the research if any further questionnaires were despatched, or if any findings from the pilot study were published. A subsequent letter (copied to the university's Vice-Chancellor) confirmed the threat. After making our apologies to the Vice-Chancellor we made our way to a meeting with the company managers.

During the 1980s the company had been involved in one of the most acrimonious industrial disputes in the history of British labour relations, which ultimately resulted in the dismissal of a substantial proportion of the striking workforce and derecognition of the trade union. The company's difficulties were further compounded when one of its ships sank in the channel, with huge loss of life. The difficulties did not end there. At the time of our pilot study, the company was introducing radical changes in staffing and rotas (which would mean that staff had to stay on board for several days without a break), and negotiating merger with its main competitor. All of these points were made clear to us in our meeting with the company managers. One of the questionnaires had found its way to Head Office where one of the Company Directors had asked why, at such a sensitive moment in the reorganization, the company was helping to provide the workforce with 'ammunition' about the relationship between work and health. The local personnel manager put the point to us bluntly: the workers could no longer contest the company's plans through the traditional mechanism of trade union negotiation, but in the wake of the shipping disaster it was felt that they might oppose the reorganization of shifts on grounds of health and safety at work. We made our apologies and left.

At the time we felt that the incident signified nothing more than an overly cautious reaction from managers facing a difficult process of reorganization. Only later did we realize that the incident was indicative of a major transformation in British labour relations which entailed the trade unions adopting a new modus operandi. At a time when trade union involvement in government policy making had been curtailed and the traditional weapons of industrial action were increasingly difficult to deploy, many trade unions were forging a new identity for themselves, increasingly focusing on the needs of individual members rather than on collective representation. This shift in emphasis included a reaffirmation of the unions' traditional role as the guardians of health and safety at work and as advocates for those made ill by their work. Concrete examples of the trade unions' role in promoting the public discourse of work stress and its consequences for health and safety at work are given in Chapter 1, but how and why did this transformation occur?

The Thatcher government's assault on trade union power during the 1980s is a central plank of the popular 'social history' of work that we outlined at the beginning of this chapter. Certainly, there is plenty of evidence to support this theme. Following the 'winter of discontent' in 1978 when the level of strike activity had reached such a point that, notoriously, the dead could not be buried, the Conservatives came to power with an overt commitment to curb the power of the unions. During the following decade five employment Acts were passed, removing the unions' blanket immunity from civil actions in tort, banning secondary picketing, ending the closed shop, and actively intervening in the way unions were run, with compulsory secret ballots for election of officers and strike action.[46] Moreover, the Thatcher government effectively closed the period of state corporatism, during which trade union leaders had been seen as essential partners (along with managers and government) in the development of economic and social policy – as Mrs Thatcher memorably put it, the union leaders would no longer be invited for 'beer and sandwiches at number ten'.

Repugnance at trade union power has a long history in Conservative Party circles. As early as 1958 the Inns of Court Conservative and Unionist Society published a pamphlet attacking the privileged legal position of the unions.[47] Memories of the role of the National Union of Mineworkers in toppling the Heath government of 1974, coupled with public frustration during the 'winter of discontent', gave further impetus to those in the party who wanted to tackle the unions. However, the demise of trade union power was not exclusively a product of the Conservatives' legislative programme.

The voluntarist tradition of British trade unionism, in which conflicts between labour and capital were largely conducted without recourse to the state, had been eroded since the mid-1960s, with the state playing an increasing role not just in protecting the rights of individual workers, but also in attempting to regulate union activities.

A central strategy was to coopt the unions into a tripartite relationship with employers and the state, in which unions would have a greater say in government but lose much of their independence. In 1969 the Labour government published a White Paper – *In Place of Strife* – which foreshadowed many of the constraints on the trade unions that would later be enshrined in the Conservative employment legislation of the 1980s. The proposals contained in the White Paper, and the more extensive constraints contained in the 1971 Industrial Relations Act (brought in by the newly elected Conservative government), were successfully opposed, or, in effect, ignored, by unions and employers alike.

During the Heath government (1970–74) the relationship between the Labour Party and the unions improved and Labour's return to office in 1974 saw a return to state corporatism with the 'social contract'. Initially this brought concessions for the unions, not least in the repeal of the Industrial Relations Act, but the economic crisis of 1975 obliged the government to implement an incomes policy which the TUC reluctantly supported. The following year brought additional austerity measures, including a £1 billion cut in public expenditure. As the economic crisis deepened the government in effect abandoned the tripartite corporatist strategy and turned to monetarist policies which placed the interests of the private sector above those of the unions. The social contract was effectively dead, and although the TUC reluctantly accepted the government's measures it was unable to hold back the tide of rank and file militancy that resulted in the 'winter of discontent'.

Thus, although the 1970s are seen as the high-water mark of union power, and the Thatcher government as its nemesis, the cooption of the trade unions, their exposure to regulation by the state and their marginalization from effective political power were all in place before the Conservatives took office in 1979.[48] Moreover, the rapid decline in union power after that date was not entirely a function of the government's legislation. The manufacturing and extractive industries which had provided the mass blue-collar membership of trade unionism, characterized by strong bonds of solidarity and a tradition of militancy, continued to decline rapidly, while the poorly unionized service sector expanded. Private sector manufacturing and extraction employed 38 per cent of the workforce in 1980, but only 25 per cent in 1998; employment in the private service sector, by contrast, grew from 26 per cent to 44 per cent over the same period.[49] Even without the legislative onslaught of a hostile Conservative government, the accompanying process of deindustrialization meant that by the beginning of the 1980s the unions were facing an uphill struggle to maintain their membership and influence.[50]

The demise of the unions over the next two decades has been rigorously charted in the series of Workplace Industrial Relations Surveys (WIRS) conducted in 1980, 1984, 1990 and 1998.[51] Trade union membership grew rapidly during the 1970s, but this trend was reversed after 1980, with aggregate union membership density for all workplaces falling from 65 per cent in that year down to 36 per cent in 1998. The decline was particularly marked in the private sector where well over half (56 per cent) of the workforce had been union members in 1980, but only a quarter were by 1998. The decline in trade union membership was matched by an equally dramatic fall in the percentage of workplaces with union recognition for collective pay bargaining. In the 1970s union leaders had brokered pay deals not just for individual workplaces, but across industries. By 1998 the percentage of workplaces recognizing unions for collective bargaining had fallen to 42 per cent, from a high of 65 per cent in 1980. And in the private sector the decline was even steeper, from 50 per cent to 25 per cent. Even where unions maintained a formal involvement in pay negotiations their bargaining power was diminished, leading the WIRS researchers to conclude: 'The system of pay determination in Britain changed over the course of our survey series from one of predominantly joint regulation to one of unilateral determination by employers or managers.'[52]

The percentage of unionized workplaces experiencing industrial action also declined, from a high of 31 per cent in 1984 down to just 4 per cent in 1998. The WIRS team suggest that industrial action is an ambiguous indicator of union strength, because strong unions can enforce their claims without resort to it. However, given the historical context this is a difficult thesis to sustain, particularly when the industrial disputes that did take place during this period are considered. Not all trade unionists eschewed militancy under the Thatcher governments; the miners, the Liverpool dockers, the print workers at Wapping and the ferry workers are just a few of the groups that fought bitter industrial disputes. However, rather than reinforcing union power such disputes only served to demonstrate the extent to which the balance of power had decisively swung in favour of the employers and the state.

The miners' strike of 1984–85 was particularly symbolic. In 1974 the miners had demonstrated that rank and file militancy was not only capable of winning industrial disputes, but also of playing a role in the toppling of governments. A decade later the contrast could not have been more pronounced. Rather than supporting the miners, the leaders of the labour movement were at best equivocal and at worst openly critical. Nightly news reports of violent clashes between strikers and the police alienated public opinion. In the early 1970s employers had been reluctant to use the measures implemented in the 1971 Employment Act, but during the 1984–85 strike the full force of the law was brought to bear through the police and the judiciary. Over the course of the dispute an important cultural transition occurred, even among supporters. At the beginning of the dispute the miners were confident of winning; placards and badges made assertive militant demands: 'Coal not dole', 'Victory to the miners'. But by the time of their eventual defeat the mood and the slogans had changed: 'Dig deep for the miners', 'Don't let them starve'. Rather than the image of the self-confident, politically conscious rank and file militant, the striking miners had become victims and charity cases. Attention shifted away from picketing and demands towards the support groups organized by miners' wives, and the effects that the defeat would have on traditional working-class communities.

In this sense, the miners' strike symbolized a major turning point in the history of British trade unionism. Its significance lies not in the loss of a particular dispute, but in the extent to which it demonstrated that workers could no longer successfully pursue their demands and defend their interests through mass strike action. Other strikes followed, but they were essentially a rerun of the same story and only served to reaffirm the belief that the old strategies could no longer succeed.

The organizational defeat of trade union militancy coincided with a major ideological shift in working-class politics. For most of the twentieth century the British labour movement had at least paid lip service to various strands of socialist ideology. At the margins this ideology was overtly anti-capitalist and revolutionary, and even among the leadership there was a degree of commitment to the social democratic agenda of using the trade unions, nationalization, Keynesian economics and statutory regulation to protect workers from the social and distributive consequences of unrestricted capitalism. In the 1950s and 1960s it was widely assumed that government had such extensive control over economic and social policy that the struggle to transform capitalism was effectively over. In *The Future of Socialism*, published in 1956, Anthony Crossland, one of the Labour Party's chief ideologues, made the following points:

> First, certain decisive sources and levers of economic power have been transferred from private business to other hands; and new levers have emerged, again concentrated in other hands than theirs. Secondly, the outcome of clashes of group or class economic interests is markedly less favourable to private employers than it used to be. Thirdly, the social attitudes and behaviour of the business class have undergone a significant change, which appears to reflect a pronounced loss of strength and self-confidence.[53]

The extent of this transformation was felt to be so great, Crossland claimed, that 'by 1951 Britain had, in all essentials, ceased to be a cap-italist country',[54] and that 'One cannot imagine today a deliberate offens-ive alliance between Government and employers against the Unions . . . or, say, a serious attempt to enforce a coal policy to which the miners bitterly objected.[55] Even at the time Crossland's optimism was attacked by critics on the left. However, our point is not that history has made a fool of Crossland, but how grossly anachronistic his views sound today and how rapidly belief in a viable socialist alternative to capitalism has withered.

By the mid-1990s the belief that capitalism could be transformed, or even tamed, by an alternative economic strategy had been expunged from the mainstream of political debate. The defeat of the unions, the demise of the Greater London Council's 'council communism', the collapse of communism across the USSR and its East European satellites, the expulsion from the Labour Party of the Militant Tendency, Tony Benn's failed bid for the party leadership, the abandonment of Clause 4 of the Labour Party's constitution (promising to secure for workers the full fruits of their labour), and the eventual creation of New Labour all reinforced Mrs Thatcher's claim that 'there is no alternative' to unrestrained free-market capitalism. Academics have reinforced the claim. In his book, *The End of History*, Francis Fukuyama has argued that the free market and liberal democracy lie at the end point of historical development and cannot be improved upon.[56] This belief is so deeply embedded in contemporary political discourse that even when critics of New Labour accuse Tony Blair of 'abandoning socialism' they are usually referring to his reluctance to put up income tax for the rich in order to fund greater public spending, rather than to the belief that there is an alternative to capitalism.

Given their tendency to focus on the pragmatic issues of pay and working conditions, the 'death of socialism' may appear to have little bearing on the role of the trade unions. However, it left the unions without an ideological basis for opposing the economic logic of late capitalism. The acceptance that there is no viable alternative to the free market necessarily entails a commitment to increased productivity, lowering of costs, flexible working and other aspects of the new managerialism, in order to compete in global markets. In short, it entails adopting much of the managerial perspective, leaving little room for a collective struggle for substantially better pay and working conditions. In this sense by the end of the 1980s British trade unionism really had become a 'hollow shell',[57] not just because of the formal constraints on their power, but because they could offer no strategic alternative to the logic of the managerial agenda.

The more prescient unions recognized the changed climate early in the 1980s. The Electrical, Electronic, Telecommunication and Plumbing Union (EETPU), was among the first to enter into single union agreements which often entailed no strike deals, acceptance of flexible working and binding arbitration.[58] The so-called 'New Realism' of moderation and concessions to employers permeated the union movement from the TUC down. As well as a retreat from confrontation and old left politics the New Realism also entailed the adoption of a more individualized relationship with union members. The managerial innovations (described above) of teamwork, performance-related pay, multi-skilling etc. meant that many workers, particularly in new sectors of the economy, increasingly related to their employers on an individual basis, personally negotiating pay, conditions and other aspects of work, rather than seeing themselves as part of a homogeneous mass of workers with the same interests and collective arrangements for negotiation. Many unions responded to such changes by offering members a more individualized form of representation, as an EETPU official noted:

We provide defence for the individual. Trade unions are giving individual advice much more on legal issues and dismissals. We are supporting the individual rather than the collective. We have the same members, we are just servicing smaller groups. It does make our job harder because we have an increasing number of calls on our time, but increasingly we are selling our services to the individual . . . For example, if you read our membership services document, we are recruiting the individual. It is all about convincing the individual we provide for them.[59]

Arguably, the New Realism has served unions and their members no better than the old militancy.[60] However, what it did do was give additional impetus to the individuation of problems at work. In a world where the apparatus of collective struggle has been dismantled and the socialist project of transforming relations at work has been abandoned, the frustrations, antagonisms and inequities of everyday working life are increasingly likely to be 'recognized' as personal grievances. If redress is to be sought, it is likely to be through the employer's grievance procedure (or failing that, through an industrial tribunal or court case), in which the trade union role is to provide advocacy, information on rights and entitlements and if necessary financial support to cover legal costs. However, the scope for grievance claims and litigation is quite limited; the employee must demonstrate that the employer has acted unfairly or illegally within the framework of policies and laws which are themselves framed within the managerial logic of late capitalism. Workers can seek redress if they are treated in a discriminatory way, or if their employer's actions contravene basic legal standards such as the minimum wage, limits on the length of the working week (a right which employees can waive), or health and safety regulations. However, there is a world of difference between an individual's entitlement to the minimum wage and the collective pursuit of an increased pay award, or opposition to redundancies. The vast range of grievances that could be explained under the 'them and us' ideology of the old labour movement, and collectively contested through mechanisms such as the strike or the 'go-slow', fit poorly into individualized managerial and juridical procedures.

One exception to this is in the area of Health and Safety at Work (HSW). Not only is the category sufficiently amorphous to include a wide range of work-related problems, it also provides a bridge between the concerns of the individual worker and the collective interests of the workforce as a whole. However, for traditional problems at work to become 'legitimate' HSW issues they must be transformed into 'causes' of physical or mental harm to the worker. The concept of 'stress' is essential to this transformation. Thus, oppressive management must become 'bullying' or 'harassment', exploitation must become 'excessive demands' or 'unreasonable pressure'. Having 'proven' that such problems can damage the health of individual workers (often through individual cases of litigation and early retirements

on medical grounds), a case can then be made for changing the workplace
to avoid further cases; a kind of HSW 'preventive medicine'.

When collective demands of this kind are presented through the medicalized prism of HSW, they take on a moral and legal impetus which is very
difficult for employers to resist. Claims which are legitimated by reference
to socialist ideology backed up by the threat of trade union militancy are
these days easily rebutted, but what employer can say that he is prepared to
risk or neglect the health and safety of his workers? Even the most laissez-
faire liberal would have difficulty justifying a return to the early nineteenth-
century model of capitalism where the health of the worker was widely
considered to be dispensable. It is these qualities of broad applicability,
relevance to individual workers, the collective dimension, and the strong
moral and legal imperative that make HSW such an attractive agenda for
contemporary trade unions.

By the end of the 1980s trade unionism may have been a 'hollow shell',
but it was a shell nonetheless; that is, it continued to exist as a set of
institutions, a membership (albeit diminished), a corpus of paid and unpaid
officials, and a sum of financial resources, even if its traditional purpose
and modus operandi were much diminished. The New Realism with its
accent on individual representation and member services (including the provision of cut price car insurance and union credit cards) partially filled this
vacuum, providing the unions with a role that went beyond that of rubber-
stamping pay deals dictated by management. HSW became an important
component of this new role, not just providing practical activities for union
officials at all levels from the workplace health and safety representative
up to the TUC advising the Health and Safety Executive, but also providing
a means of addressing some of the old collective concerns in a form which
employers and even Conservative governments could hardly oppose. Thus,
while virtually every other aspect of trade union power was diminished
during the 1980s, the number of HSW committees remained constant. Commenting on their series of Workplace Industrial Relations Surveys, Millward
et al. conclude: 'The only structures for collective employee voice that we
found to be as common in 1998 as they had been in 1980 were health and
safety committees.'[61]

The increasing centrality of HSW to modern trade unions goes some
way to explaining their vigorous promotion of the public discourse of work
stress and their involvement in high-profile court cases, as described in
Chapter 1.

To summarize the changes that took place in the British trade union movement between the late 1970s and mid-1990s: the formal union involvement
in government policy making that had characterized state corporatism
in the 1970s was brought to a close; large-scale collective bargaining was
increasingly replaced by locally (or individually) negotiated agreements,
particularly in the private sector; legislation curtailed many of the immunities

and rights, particularly regarding the closed shop, secondary picketing and internal affairs; membership and militancy both declined rapidly; the socialist or social democratic agenda that had previously been posited as an alternative strategy to neo-liberalism collapsed and was replaced by a largely uncritical New Realism; collective representation was increasingly replaced by individualized services, such as advocacy; and concerns about HSW became an important mechanism through which traditional concerns were expressed. But what effect might these changes have had on the experiences of workers, and how did they contribute to the rise of the work stress phenomenon?

First, it can be argued that the collapse of trade union power left workers operationally incapable of defending themselves against the onslaught of neo-liberal economic and social policies which reduced many of the welfare concessions granted in the post-war settlement, and the flexibilization and intensification of the labour process that accompanied the new managerialism. From this perspective, the balance of power shifted decisively in favour of employers who were able to push workers harder – some would argue, to the point of psychological and physical breakdown. This line of argument is persuasive, but does it fully explain the work stress phenomenon? Trade union power has collapsed before, during the 1930s,[62] but there is no evidence of a subsequent work stress epidemic. Also, as we discussed above, although there is evidence that the labour process intensified after 1980, the apparent increase in job insecurity and length of the working week may have been overstated and even the increase in work effort seems relatively modest when compared with earlier periods. Moreover, if employers really were bent on squeezing more out of their workers, one would expect wages to remain static or even decrease as productivity increased, but work intensification in Europe has been accompanied by rising real wages.[63] While the ability of unions to defend their members' interests appears to have diminished, the evidence suggests that this may only be a partial explanation of why the work stress epidemic emerged at this time.

A second approach to the relationship between the changing face of trade unions and the rise of the work stress phenomenon, which looks at the discursive significance, is arguably more convincing. The discursive impact that the changing face of trade unionism has had on the consciousness of workers is twofold. Coupled with the collapse of socialist and social democratic ideologies, the transition to New Realism in which unions take on board the economic and managerial logic of late capitalism has robbed workers of the belief that the social organization and structure of work could be viably transformed. There have been other moments in the historical development of the capitalist mode of production when employers have had the upper hand and workers have been virtually powerless to resist their demands, but on all these earlier occasions the possibility has always remained that the labour movement would one day redress the balance. The absolute disappearance of socialist utopias has imbued contemporary forms of work with an appearance of immutability. In a world in which it is assumed that 'there is no alternative' to neo-liberal economics and the new management, it is not surprising that workers should begin to internalize adverse experiences at work, seeing them as personal problems of coping and adaptation rather than collective questions of power and alienation.

The reorientation of the unions towards the HSW agenda can only reinforce this tendency, effectively medicalizing experiences which in an earlier period might have been interpreted as grounds for industrial action. Not only does this process influence what course of action is taken (sick leave, counselling, medication, retirement on medical grounds, litigation); it may also shape the way in which embodied emotional states are interpreted – boredom becomes despair, dissatisfaction becomes depression, anger becomes anxiety, the physiological changes (triggered by the autonomic nervous system) that prepare the body to fight become the precursors of heart disease.

Changes in the character of work and the trade unions go some way to explaining why adverse experiences at work have become depoliticized and individualized; however, there are broader cultural changes outside the workplace that have also contributed to this process and which further explain why the work stress phenomenon has taken a particular medicalized form. It is to these broader cultural influences that we now turn.

The changing state of emotions

'Pull yourself together', 'Get a grip', 'Chin up', 'Stiff upper lip', 'Don't let the bastards grind you down.' These folk incitements to resilience, familiar enough to a wartime generation that endured the blitz and rationing, have not only gone out of fashion, they have become grossly insensitive and politically incorrect. For liberal commentators they are considered to be emblematic of 'old England', an age of repression when human feelings were denied or subjected to a Victorian code of discipline and restraint, exemplified by the quasi-militarist regime of the public school. This caricature of old England is frequently contrasted with the new progressive age of emotional enlightenment, characterized by more open (and often public) expression of feelings, greater sensitivity to people's emotional needs and mental vulnerability, and the provision of informal and statutory forms of support and therapy to help individuals to cope with the stresses and strains of everyday life. For many commentators this transition is not just cultural, but political – 'stiff upper lip' is conservative, expressive emotionality is progressive.

The politicization of emotional life is nowhere more apparent than in the think tank 'Antidote', backed by many of New Labour's most prominent supporters including Glenys Kinnock, Patricia Hewitt, Helena Kennedy,

David Puttnam, and the social theorist Anthony Giddens.[64] The aim of Antidote is to generate greater 'emotional literacy' by bringing psychological insights to bear on virtually all aspects of public policy.[65] One of the founders of Antidote, Andrew Samuels, has recently argued that a psychotherapist should sit on all government policy committees and that the emotional and spiritual effects of policy proposals should be constantly monitored.[66]

In Chapter 3 we discussed the sociology of emotions and the concept of 'feeling rules', that is, the set of informal beliefs and social conventions that govern emotional behaviour, for example that it is not appropriate to laugh during funerals. As well as guiding our behaviour these rules also influence our subjectivity and sense of self. These feeling rules and the subjectivities they give rise to are culturally and historically specific. Thus, it is possible to identify a particular 'ethnopsychology', that comprises the sum of rules and beliefs about human subjectivity, personhood, and emotional life.[67] Medical discourse, particularly concerning mental health, plays a central role in shaping these cultural expectations. As Derek Summerfield has suggested, the diagnostic categories of psychiatry have a powerful influence on the way in which individuals make sense of their experiences, and on their future behaviour:

> The constructs of 'psychology' or 'mental health' are social products. Collectively held beliefs about particular negative experiences are not just potent influences but carry an element of self-fulfilling prophecy; individuals will largely organize what they say, feel, do, and expect to fit prevailing expectations and categories. Underpinning these constructs is the concept of 'person' that is held by a particular culture at a particular point in time. This embodies questions such as how much or what kind of adversity a person can face and still be 'normal'; what is reasonable risk; when fatalism is appropriate and when a sense of grievance is; what is acceptable behaviour at a time of crisis including how distress should be expressed, how help should be sought, and whether restitution should be made.[68]

Tracking these transitions in the ethnopsychology presents a methodological difficulty. When we discussed changes in the world of work there were at least some 'objective' data on which to hang the analysis, for example time series data on job tenure and hours worked per week, even if these data were sometimes misleading or difficult to interpret. But changes in cultural norms of personhood and emotionality are even harder to quantify because of their deeply subjective character. We may intuitively feel that the tradition of British stoicism – the stiff upper lip – has been eroded, but how can we demonstrate this empirically?

Our strategy is twofold. In the remainder of this chapter we will attempt to grasp changes in the ethnopsychology by discourse analysis, focusing on three key emergent discursive formations: the vulnerable body; victim culture;

and the therapeutic state. There are two problems with this approach. First, it might be dismissed as 'impressionistic', i.e. that we are simply selecting evidence that reinforces our thesis and ignoring that which contradicts it. A second criticism is that changes in discourse may not be reflected in the consciousness of individuals. To combat these criticisms we return, in the final chapter, to a qualitative analysis of the extent to which these putative cultural changes are reflected in the consciousness of individuals, specifically in relation to their beliefs and experiences regarding therapeutic interventions for work stress.

Vulnerable bodies

In the developed world most objective indicators of health improved rapidly throughout the last century. Infant mortality fell from 142 per 1000 live births in 1901 to 6.2 per thousand by the end of the 1990s, and life expectancy at birth rose from 45.5 years for men and 49 years for women to 74.4 years for men and 79.7 years for women over the same period. Infectious diseases such as cholera, typhoid, measles, whooping cough, tuberculosis, diphtheria, and poliomyelitis, which were widespread in the Victorian period, are now a rarity. As more people survived into old age the number of people dying from cancers, heart disease and strokes increased, but even so the British public can now expect to live longer, healthier lives than at any previous time in their history.[69]

Yet despite continuing improvements in health, British society is obsessed with health scares and panics, many of which pose little threat or are based on extremely slender or non-existent evidence. Michael Fitzpatrick has produced a compelling analysis of health scares and the evidence behind them, including major panics about HIV/AIDS, cot death, malignant moles, oral contraceptives, the human form of mad cow disease, MMR and autism; and minor ones about necrotizing fasciitis, drug-resistant superbugs, electromagnetic fields, silicone breast implants, nuclear power, salmonella in eggs, and water and air pollution.[70] The list could be extended, as virtually every week stories can be found in the press linking seemingly innocuous substances and activities to disease and early death. Literally on the day that this paragraph was written the *Guardian* newspaper reported that EU scientists were calling for an urgent review of the safety of hair dyes following the publication of US research suggesting that use of permanent hair dyes could double or treble the risk of contracting bladder cancer.[71]

Much of the 'evidence' on which health scares are based is questionable,[72] leading one commentator to suggest that the public interest would best be served by the closure of university departments of epidemiology.[73] And even the most prominent health scares, such as those concerning HIV/AIDS, vCJD, MMR, and oral contraceptive pills, have often provoked an equally high-profile backlash frequently promoted by experts in the field questioning the empirical evidence. However, as Fitzpatrick (writing of his experiences as a general practitioner) has observed, a backlash of this kind is rarely sufficient to allay public fears:

> It is, of course, still possible to have sex without a condom, but as numerous patients have told me, it is not easy to remove from the back of the mind the worry that this might result in a lethal contamination. It is no longer possible to put a baby in a cot without thinking about which way round they should be lying ... People still lie in the sun on those rare occasions it appears in Britain's cloudy skies, but not without applying their sunscreen cream ... Women still take the Pill, but now in a state of heightened awareness of a risk of sudden death from thrombosis ... The proportion of meat eaters has never returned to the level before the mad cow scare ... Most parents still choose to have their babies vaccinated against measles, mumps and rubella, but none now without a twinge of anxiety that this may destine them to a devastating disability.[74]

Many people are selective about which health scares to act upon and which to ignore and there are many lay strategies for defusing the impact of health promotion imperatives – the token tub of low fat spread at the back of the fridge; tales of 'Uncle Norman' who survived to a ripe old age on 80 cigarettes a day.[75-6] Yet despite these strategies the health scares of the 1980s and 1990s have given rise to a heightened sense of physical vulnerability.

Londoners may breathe cleaner air than they did in the 1950s, the water we drink may be purer than at any point in our history, the variety and quality of our food may dramatically exceed that of the third world, medical science may offer treatments for many of our ills, but the belief that the mundane activities of everyday life – eating, drinking, making love, breathing city air, lying in the sun – may lead to an early death has never been more deeply embedded in the public consciousness. In a world where a relationship is posited between events as prosaic as dyeing one's hair and dying of cancer, or drinking coffee and succumbing to heart disease, it is hardly surprising that the equally banal experiences of working life should take on the appearance of pathological agents. If the body is vulnerable to sunshine or sex, then why not to a heavy workload or a bullying boss? This conclusion is reinforced by the perception that the body is not only highly vulnerable to cancers and cardiovascular disease, but also to psychiatric and emotional pathologies.

In the early 1990s the mental health charity SANE ran a poster campaign bearing the slogan 'You don't have to be mentally ill to suffer from a mental illness.' At first sight the slogan appears paradoxical, but, as with all good advertisements, a closer reading reveals a wealth of meaning. The underlying message is that it is not just the social stereotypes of the danger-ous schizophrenic or suicidal depressive that have mental health problems; 'ordinary' people, like the reader of the poster, may also suffer psychological problems which might benefit from formal or informal support. Mental health is reconceptualized as a continuum rather than a strict dichotomy between the sane and the mad. The intention is to remove the stigma of mental illness, for two reasons; first, to remove the alterity or 'otherness' of those with severe problems in order to reduce discrimination against them, and secondly, to encourage those with comparatively minor problems to seek help.

The themes expressed in the SANE poster campaign are deeply embedded in the post-war history of British mental health care including the gradual closure of the large Victorian asylums, the rather parsimonious transition to care in the community, and the growth of patients' rights. Many of these developments were motivated, at least rhetorically, by humanist beliefs about the rights and dignity of the mentally ill. Rather than being treated as social pariahs, the mentally ill were to be recognized as human beings, entitled to the respect and support of the community. Given this emphasis it is profoundly ironic that the conception of mental illness as a continuous rather than dichotomous variable has had such a profoundly anti-humanist effect by lowering social expectations of mental resilience and emotional competence.

Blurring the distinction between severe mental illness and the adverse emotional experiences of everyday life may have been motivated by a desire to improve the lot of the mentally ill, but it has had the adverse con-sequence of increasing our sense of mental or psychological vulnerability. The number of categories of 'abnormal behaviour' recognized by the Amer-ican Psychiatric Association rose from 60 in 1952 to 384 in 1994.[77] The expansion of psychiatric categories has permeated virtually every aspect of emotional and psychological life. Naughty children may be suffering from Attention Deficit Hyperactivity Disorder; people who eat too little (or too much) may have an eating disorder; post-Christmas gloominess may be a symptom of Seasonal Affective Disorder caused by lack of sunlight (this last one is difficult to square with the threat of skin cancer – clearly a diffi-cult balance must be struck). Emotional problems that might previously have been considered a 'normal' response to everyday life are increasingly redefined as symptoms of mental illness.

A central theme of the psychiatrization of everyday life is the claim that our feelings and behaviour are determined by factors that lie outside our personal control.[78] Thus, the categories of addiction and codependency are employed to 'explain' an ever-increasing range of excessive behaviours and activities, from smoking, drinking alcohol and using recreational drugs through to playing video games, gambling on the national lottery, or even (as the case of film star Michael Douglas brought to the public eye) having lots of sex. The common theme is that such 'addicts' have been exposed to a substance or experience that has rendered them incapable of exercising rational control over their behaviour:

> The ideal of the self-determining individual has given way to a more diminished interpretation of subjectivity and the pathology of addiction provides a new standard for determining behaviour.[79]

Closely related to these themes of addiction and the diminished self is the concept of 'trauma' which suggests that exposure to adverse experiences can leave 'emotional scars' from which the individual may never recover. The category of post-traumatic stress disorder (PTSD) has its origins in the aftermath of the American war in Vietnam as a way of relating the psychological problems of veterans to their experiences of atrocities committed against Vietnamese peasants by the US military.[80] Initially the diagnosis was limited to extreme experiences such as war or major disasters, but it quickly spread to more commonly encountered experiences; for instance, road traffic accidents have been found to be the commonest cause of PTSD.[81] Even those who are not physically injured by a traffic accident can still claim damages for PTSD; motorist Mark Cooper was awarded £476,000 in damages for the 'acute sickness, anger and flashbacks' he suffered after running over a 4-year-old girl, who later made a full recovery.[82] Indeed, 'victims' of PTSD need not have been present at the incident that provoked their problems; in the most recent edition of the *Diagnostic and Statistical Manual of Mental Disorders*, the diagnosis has been expanded to include friends and relatives who hear about the adverse experiences of their loved ones.[83] One commentator has even gone so far as suggesting that television viewers may be vulnerable to PTSD after seeing the 'televisual horror' of news reports about train crashes and other disasters.[84] The broadening scope of the diagnosis has been matched by an explosion of academic publications, with 16,000 indexed by 1999.[85]

Given the wide range of experiences that are claimed to give rise to PTSD it is not surprising that the phenomenon has also arisen in the work setting. Salad bar manager Stephen Rickard took his employer Sainsbury's to an industrial tribunal after they sacked him for taking four months sick leave allegedly caused by PTSD following an incident in which some of his customers contracted dysentery.[86] Even highly trained professionals in the public services, who presumably expect to encounter distressing events in the course of their working lives, have not proved immune to PTSD. In financial terms the claims made by professionals attending disasters can often outstrip those of the actual victims; for example, more than a decade after the Hillsborough football stadium disaster, a retired police sergeant was awarded £330,000 for the 'late-onset' PTSD he claimed to have suffered as a result – a sum 100 times greater than that awarded to the families of fans who had died at the match.[87] Similarly, victims' groups were angered when a prison warder won £150,000 in compensation for the 'psychological horrors' brought on by counselling child sex offenders – victims of sex crimes can receive a maximum of £33,000 in compensation from the criminal injuries compensation authority.[88]

Central to the PTSD category is the belief that exposure to emotionally disturbing events is equivalent to a physical injury; that our emotional state can be 'scarred' in the same way that the flesh can be disfigured. The implication is that individuals have no control over the extent of their 'injury'; they are simply passive victims of events. Similarly, it is deemed unlikely that PTSD sufferers will be able to 'heal' themselves without recourse to professional intervention, either through 'talking cures' such as cognitive behaviour therapy or more unusually through the administration of stress hormones such as hydrocortisone.[89] Thus, in many major (or even comparatively minor) traumatic incidents it is common practice for the stress counsellors to be despatched almost before the ambulances, even though the available empirical evidence suggests that those who receive individual debriefing may fare worse than those who receive no intervention.[90]

The cultural significance of the rapid expansion of mental illness categories, addictions and emotional trauma is not just that they diminish the role of subjectivity in governing behaviour, but that (like the physical health scares described above) they give a heightened sense of vulnerability. The impression is that the mind as well as the body can be easily damaged by the experiences we encounter in everyday life, and that the extent of the damage is likely to exceed our ability to cope without professional help.

Frank Furedi has illustrated the cultural change that has occurred in expectations of emotional resilience in his analysis of the Aberfan coal tip disaster.[91] On October 21 1966, 116 schoolchildren and 28 adults were killed when tons of coal slurry slipped down a hill and buried their school. Despite the horrific nature of the incident none of the villagers sought compensation, surviving children returned to school two weeks after the disaster and a child psychologist appraising the children a year later found them to be normal and well-adjusted. Furedi contrasts the stoicism of the Aberfan families against the likely response in the current climate:

> Today such a response to a major disaster would be unthinkable. There would be an automatic assumption that every survivor in the area was deeply traumatized and inevitably scarred for life. Sending young pupils back to school so soon after a tragedy would be scorned as bad practice. The very attempt by the community to cope through self help would be denounced as misguided since such victims could not be expected to deal with such problems on their own.[92]

However, even long past events can be reinterpreted to fit in with contemporary assumptions and the Welsh Office has recently funded an £80,000 research project to be conducted by a team from Cardiff University's College of Medicine which will ask survivors to give details of 'any psychological problems they have experienced – including everything from drug and alcohol use to depression and post-traumatic stress disorder'. Jeff Edwards, a survivor rescued from an air pocket beneath the mud, was equivocal about the new research: 'I welcome the new research, but not all the survivors will agree. There are still people who will not talk about their experience, and this research will rake up unwanted memories.'[93]

The heightened sense of mental and physical vulnerability described above has created a tendency to interpret emotionally distressing experiences and personal hardships in terms of medical and psychiatric categories and this has played a fundamental role in the genesis of the current work stress epidemic. Whatever the extent of actual changes in the demands and pressures placed on workers, their ability to withstand and resist such pressures has been sapped by the cultural retreat from resilience. It is not just the possibility of a substantial compensation pay-out that has brought about this change (only a small minority of those who lay claim to the work stress identity receive such sums). Another contributing factor is the way in which the identity of 'victim' has achieved a new moral authority and high social status.

Victim culture

Nothing exemplifies the cult of the victim more than the life and premature death of Diana, Princess of Wales. Unprecedented scenes of public grief followed her fatal car accident in September 1997. Within hours of the announcement crowds gathered outside the gates of Kensington Palace, depositing a pile of flowers so vast that it eventually had to be cleared with a bulldozer. As well as interviews with Diana's friends and associates (indeed, anyone remotely acquainted with her), the constant media coverage also carried reports and images of 'a nation united in grief'. Men and women who had no connection with the princess and had never met her were filmed literally sobbing in the street and declaiming the extent to which she had touched their lives and the deep sense of personal loss that they felt. In the days that followed the funeral the public mood was contrasted with the rather staid response of the royal household and it was suggested that the absence of a more expressive display of grief might have damaged the monarchy.

The contrast with the dignified mourning of earlier public figures could not have been more pronounced. The tradition of British reserve and stoicism had been replaced by a new accent on demonstrativeness and open pronouncements of emotional suffering. We have already described the new emotionality, but in this instance the phenomenon was very much related to events in Diana's life and her efforts, despite a lifetime of wealth and privilege, to present herself as a universal victim. In a televised interview with Martin Bashir, broadcast shortly before her death, Diana described intimate details of her loveless marriage to Charles, her abuse by the royal household, her betrayal by former lover James Hewitt, and her eventual collapse into bulimia and attempted suicide. Asked if she still wanted to be queen, Diana replied that she wanted to be 'the queen of people's hearts' and that she saw her new role as an emotional ambassador for Britain. The suggestion was that her personal experiences of emotional distress, coupled with her patronage of various charitable causes, including visits to AIDS sufferers and the homeless, had enabled her to understand the needs of victims and to act as their advocate. In laying claim to the identity of victim, Diana was doing more than staking out a new role for herself; she was demanding the high moral status, public sympathy/empathy and privileged voice that such an identity confers. That she was subsequently 'hounded to death by the tabloids' put the final seal on her claim to victimhood.

In adopting the identity of 'victim' as a moral claim for public support and a privileged voice Diana was utilizing (and contributing to) a broader cultural shift. A key component of victim culture concerns social recognition and validation; this is particularly evident in the field of criminal justice. During the 1960s criminologists pointed to the disparity between official crime statistics based on crimes reported to police and the 'dark figure of unreported crime' gleaned from self-report surveys.[94] The suggestion was that many of the victims of crime were suffering in silence with their needs ignored by society. Sociology with its traditional focus on the criminal or 'deviant' was itself vulnerable to this charge, as reflected in a joke that was in circulation at the time. In a variation on the parable of the Good Samaritan, a man lies in the street beaten and robbed. The first passer by crosses the street to avoid involvement, but then two sociologists come along. They approach the man and he tells them what has happened to him, and one sociologist turns to the other and says, 'Whoever did this needs our help.' The subdiscipline of 'victimology' was born in response.

The belief in a large pool of silent victims rapidly spread from criminal justice to other domains and has become a ubiquitous theme among those making claims on behalf of others. The recent report by the British Medical Association (BMA) on domestic violence illustrates the spread of victimology and the extent to which vicarious claims making of this kind often entails statistical manipulation.[95] Most people might assume that domestic violence entails physical or sexual abuse; however the BMA's definition also includes verbal and psychological abuse, including criticism. Widening the definition in this way grossly inflates the prevalence rate, enabling the BMA to claim that one in four women will be victims of domestic violence at some point in their lives. The BMA report also cited a Canadian survey of general practitioners in which over half the respondents believed that they were missing 30 per cent or more cases of domestic violence. As Fitzpatrick has observed,

'Such GPs, who can estimate the percentage of an unknown quantity, are wasted in general practice (though they might find a successful career in epidemiology).'[96]

Since the 1960s social scientists and professional groups have played an important role in placing victimhood on the public agenda; however, victim support groups have also contributed to the politicization of victimhood. Support groups can now be found for virtually any adverse experience or hardship,[97] including survivors of child abuse, domestic violence, bullying at school and at work, sexual harassment, even second- or third-generation concentration camp victims (the children or grandchildren of holocaust victims whose lives have been affected by their relatives' experiences). Such groups often base themselves on the model developed by Alcoholics Anonymous, using group discussions among fellow sufferers and survivors to provide support for coping strategies. Similarly, television programmes that portray or discuss themes relating to victims often provide a telephone advice line for the benefit of viewers whose concerns or anxieties have been aroused. However, some victim support groups have organized themselves as pressure groups to lobby for political change. Such groups often seek legitimacy by arguing that their experiences give them a privileged insight into the nature of a particular problem and the moral authority to demand change. For instance, Diana Lamplugh, whose estate agent daughter Suzy was murdered in the course of her work, became a prominent 'public safety expert' giving advice to policy makers.

Such efforts often reflect a desire to give symbolic meaning to inherently meaningless experiences of suffering and death, to support the claim that a victim has not suffered in vain.[98] In the United States, Megan's Law was introduced to reveal the identity and address of sex offenders, after 7-year-old Megan Kanka of New Jersey was raped and murdered by a neighbour whose previous convictions for sex offences had been concealed. Whereas close emotional involvement in an issue might previously have been seen as a disqualification from the supposedly rational policy-making process, it is increasingly seen as an essential component, as if the experience of suffering gives a special insight into how a social problem might be resolved – an effective trump card over rational appraisal of effectiveness or concerns about civil liberties. Victim impact statements were proposed by Michael Howard under the Conservative government's *Victim's Charter* to enable the victims of crime to express their emotional injuries in court. Similarly, the current Labour administration is making plans for 'restorative justice' which will put the needs of the victim at the centre of the criminal justice system.

The promotion of victimhood has been allied to a corrosion of the distinction between public and private. Laying claim to the social identity of victim invariably entails the public performance of emotional disclosure. Following an abduction or murder it is common practice for the police to parade the extreme emotional distress of relatives at a press conference, presumably in the hope that witnesses or even the perpetrator will be moved to come forward. Where grief and emotional anguish were previously considered to be private matters shared at most with relatives and close friends, they are increasingly becoming objects of public scrutiny and confession. The media are strewn with first-hand accounts of the emotional effects of divorce, illness, addiction, bereavement and abuse. Political figures and celebrities are by no means immune to this tendency, and in the absence of any other adverse experiences to emote about, celebrity itself is articulated as a cause of emotional suffering because of the intrusiveness of the press or the demands of fans.

The public appetite for unmediated 'raw' emotion is so great that television companies have resorted to manufacturing it. In so called 'reality TV' shows like *Big Brother* and *Survivor*, groups of contestants are placed in an emotionally challenging environment and left to emote in front of the ever present cameras. *Big Brother* is an exercise in what might be termed the presentation of the emotional self. Success or failure depends upon the contestant's capacity to navigate the new etiquette of emotionality; displaying their emotional honesty, authenticity and personal warmth, without revealing 'negative' emotions like anger or aggression – contestants who argue are usually among the first to be evicted. The show illustrates the complicated way in which the morality of victimhood is intertwined with public displays of emotion. In the first series 'naughty Nick' pretended that his girlfriend had been killed in a car crash in order to engage the sympathy of his fellow contestants; however, claims of victimhood are only accepted if they are based on the absolute passivity of the claimant. Thus, when Nick tried to exonerate himself (from charges of cheating) by literally breaking down and blaming his character defects on a public school education and a job in the City, his plea for victim status was not accepted. Similarly, Vanessa Feltz's emotional breakdown (on the celebrity version of the show) was not accepted because her behaviour was so disturbed that it became a problem for the other members of the group – she had in effect drifted across the narrow boundary that separates victim from aggressor.

Claims of victimhood can only be made to stick if they are made by a demonstrably powerless self. By this we refer to an extremely diminished will to act, rather than to structural determinants of power such as wealth or status. Thus, Diana could successfully lay claim to victim status by demonstrating her lack of agency, despite her wealth and privilege. Embracing victimhood necessarily entails relinquishing agency. Thus, the reverse side of the incitement to victimhood is the pathologization of the active self.

This theme is readily apparent in the feminist critique of masculinity. Traditionally feminism has been concerned with achieving equality with men by challenging structural constraints, such as access to education, employment, birth control, and by challenging assumptions about women's emotional and physical frailty. From this perspective the supposedly masculine traits of self-possession, assertiveness, courage and heroism can be viewed as desirable characteristics which women are equally capable of adopting. The critique of masculinity turns this perspective on its head. Gender stereotypes are still viewed as social constructions which can be changed, but it is traditionally male characteristics which are viewed as problematic and pathological.[99-100] Male assertiveness leads to violence and crime,[101] self-possession is a form of autism, comradeship is a strategy for excluding women, and courage reveals an inability to care. The problem lies not in essential unchangeable attributes of men and women, but in the way men are socialized, i.e. the way men are brought up and the social expectations of them.[102] Rather than women aspiring to be more like men, it is argued, society must recognize that many of the attributes traditionally associated with women, such as caring and nurturing, should be valued and their development encouraged among men as well as women, while 'macho culture' should be constrained and discouraged.

Unchecked masculinity or 'machismo' is not only seen as a problem for women, but also for men, who must live up to social expectations which are psychologically damaging. Some commentators have even suggested that machismo is to blame for men's shorter life expectancy as men are more likely to take risks, engage in unhealthy activities like smoking tobacco and drinking alcohol, and are more reluctant to seek medical help, or even admit that they have health problems. One advocate of the 'men's health' movement suggests that: 'The road to improvement in men's health lies in puncturing typical myths of masculinity such as that it's good to be daring, unemotional and in control.'[103]

By identifying masculinity with aggressive anti-social and self-destructive behaviour, the critics of masculinity effectively pathologize human agency. Rather than actively engaging in the world and struggling to transform it, men and women are encouraged to retreat inside themselves, to lead more contemplative and expressive lives. This very closely mirrors the transformation in trade unionism described above. Rather than the aggressive rank and file militant of the early stage of the miners' strike, literally fighting for his rights, trade unionists are adopting a less adversarial and more individualized identity, often presenting themselves as the passive victims of bullying, uncaring management. As Kaminer has observed, it is the pathologization of agency that has led to the hymning of victimhood: 'If we valued action or believed in it, if we felt that the world was even partly of our own making, we'd treat victims with compassion and respect but not reverence.'[104]

The moral authority and privileged voice currently ascribed to victimhood make it an attractive identity for those making claims; but these advantages come at a high price – a diminished sense of agency and resilience. The discourse of work stress draws together the broad cultural changes described above, the heightened perception of mental and physical vulnerability and the moral imperatives of victimhood and combines them with changed expectations of work and trade unionism, effectively corroding resilience and the will to resist, in favour of the passive and introspective subjectivity of the work stress victim. One final cultural change which explains why the work stress phenomenon has taken a specifically medicalized form is the growth of the therapeutic state.

The therapeutic state

As we described above, the number of psychiatric categories has expanded rapidly in the post-war period to encompass an increasingly broad range of human problems and emotional difficulties; what Kramer describes as 'diagnostic bracket creep'.[105] One might expect that an expansion in the breadth of mental illness would necessarily entail a proportionate increase in the psychiatric apparatus, i.e. more psychiatrists and more psychiatric facilities. However, as Simon Wessley has observed, psychiatrists and the scarce resources available to them are increasingly ghettoized in the treatment of severe mental illness, leaving the broad field of 'non-psychotic' problems to a growing band of largely 'enthusiastic but unskilled and unsupervised' counsellors.[106] The expansion of counselling services in general medical practice was greatly enhanced by the introduction of the new GP contract in 1990 which allowed 70 per cent of the cost of employing counsellors to be reimbursed – an attractive proposition for hard-pressed GPs eager to free themselves from the emotional and relationship problems of 'heartsink' patients, and the demands of the new health promotion agenda. Thus, as well as addressing problems of anxiety, depression and relationships, counselling was also advocated for 'smoking cessation, modification of diet, alcohol misuse, post-natal depression, addiction to tranquillisers, and high-risk sexual behaviour'.[107] By the end of the 1990s over half of all general practices employed one or more counsellors, making the National Health Service the major employer of therapeutic professionals.[108]

Even more surprising than the growth of health service counselling is its equally rapid growth in education, social work, policing and probation and even commerce and industry. Counselling is a loose category, making it difficult to obtain reliable evidence of the number of full- or part-time counsellors; one estimate suggests there may be as many as 110,000, not including the vast number of teachers, lecturers, social workers, managers, doctors and nurses who see counselling as part of their job.[109]

Frank Furedi[110] suggests that the therapeutic culture has permeated the welfare state to such a degree that it now underpins virtually every public policy. For example, the poverty debate has shifted away from strategies of wealth redistribution towards more therapeutic measures aimed at raising self-esteem and reducing feelings of social exclusion.[111] Therapeutic techniques also feature in government strategies for reducing teenage pregnancies, reducing unemployment, improving parenting skills, tackling drug abuse and anti-social behaviour, child prostitution, and low educational attainment. Whatever the social ill, the solution is deemed to be a therapeutic intervention such as counselling to boost self-esteem and foster social inclusion. The adoption of a therapeutic approach to public policy has had the effect of transforming the relationship between the individual and the state. This has been achieved by blurring the boundary between the public and private domains, greatly expanding the state's capacity to intervene in virtually every aspect of a person's emotional life and relationships:

> Today, the line that divides the public from the private has become increasingly porous as public therapeutic authority arrogates for itself new responsibilities for the regulation and management of the self. The rise of therapeutic culture is inexorably linked to the reorganisation of the relationship between the public and private. Moreover by gaining a privileged role for the regulation of personal relationships, therapeutic authority can claim constant access to the private sphere.[112]

The question is, why are people not only prepared to accept this intrusion, but in some instances actively seek it out and demand it? The answer is to do with recognition and validation. In a society with a heightened sense of physical and mental vulnerability, coupled with the diminished subjectivity characterized by the agency-robbing culture of victimhood, therapeutic 'diagnosis' and 'treatment' can provide an important source of existential security. Where the threats to the self are perceived to be overwhelming and the personal emotional resources for dealing with them are felt to be inadequate, it is hardly surprising that more and more people are willing to relinquish sovereignty over their mental life and allow the agents of the therapeutic state to play an increased role in governing their behaviour and relationships. The medicalization of personal problems not only offers moral exoneration, but also a course of action; for example, the feelings of guilt and the strain of dealing with an energetically disruptive child might be eased considerably by a diagnosis of Attention Deficit Hyperactivity Disorder, and the provision of behavioural therapy or a prescription for Ritalin. As Gergen has suggested, therapeutic culture offers 'invitations to infirmity'.[113]

The strategies and apparatuses of the therapeutic state provide an answer to the problems raised by vulnerable bodies and the culture of victimhood. This has a very direct bearing on the work stress phenomenon, not least because the therapeutic apparatus is directly available in many workplaces. Stressed university lecturers are increasingly availing themselves of the stress counselling services provided for students; other universities are setting up separate services exclusively for staff who might otherwise feel stigmatized if seen attending by their students.[114] Stress helplines have been set up for doctors and teachers (see Chapter 1). When Cleveland Council was disbanded in 1995 and its employees reassigned to a reorganized local authority, 18 bereavement counsellors were appointed to advise staff that their sense of loss could be similar to the death of 'a friend or loved one' and that they should expect symptoms such as loss of libido, mood swings, eating disorders and panic attacks.[115]

Human resource management and personnel staff are becoming increasingly embroiled in the therapeutic ethos. Many of the larger private companies are not only buying in counselling services for their staff, but are training managers to use counselling skills in their work.[116] In his account of the rise of therapeutic culture in Britain, Nicholas Rose suggests that 'The management of subjectivity has become a central task for the modern organisation.'[117] Outside the workplace, the therapeutic state is so overwhelmingly pervasive that even workers who do not have direct access to counselling services at work are likely to interpret their experiences in therapeutic terms and seek help from their doctor or an NHS counsellor.

We set out to answer two questions in this chapter. Has work become harder? And has our emotional/mental resilience been eroded? In the first half of the chapter we considered empirical evidence of changes in job tenure, hours worked per week, work intensification, new managerial techniques, and changes in trade unionism. The evidence is mixed; average job tenure and the length of the working week appear to have changed little for most workers, although there is evidence to show that work intensified during the 1980s, with the introduction of flexible working, and that the balance of power in the workplace shifted away from unionized labour towards employers.

While there is some support for the argument that the Thatcher years squeezed more out of the British worker and withdrew some of the concessions granted earlier in the century, it is our contention that these changes are not sufficient to explain the emergence of the work stress epidemic. Of course there is a difficulty in moving from a macro analysis of changes in work to a micro analysis of the experiences of particular workers. And it is plausible that particular workers have encountered experiences at work that are so overwhelmingly demanding that they directly cause psychological harm without the mediation of other factors. Of course it is possible literally to work people to death through a combination of excessive fatigue, brutality and malnutrition. And while such extreme conditions are not found in British workplaces, it is possible to believe that some workers may endure excessively long hours, for minimal pay and under extremely coercive conditions, but 'slave labour' of this kind lies at the very margins of employment in Britain; it crosses into the realm of illegality.

It is extremely unlikely that a significant proportion of the British workforce are routinely being pushed beyond the limits of human endurance by their experiences at work. This becomes immediately apparent if we take a broader historical perspective and compare work today with that in earlier periods of industrialization[118] or even in the feudal period.[119] It is sometimes suggested that although contemporary work may be less physically demanding than in the past, flexible working and insecurity mean that contemporary workers face far greater psychological pressures than their forebears, but consider Eric Hobsbawm's account of work in the late nineteenth century:

> If any single factor dominated the lives of nineteenth-century workers it was insecurity. They did not know at the beginning of the week how much they would bring home at the end. They did not know how long their present job would last or, if they lost it, when they would get another job or under what conditions. They did not know when accident or sickness would hit them, and though they knew that some time in middle age – perhaps in the forties for unskilled labourers, perhaps in the fifties for the more skilled – they would become incapable of doing a full measure of adult physical labour, they did not know what would happen to them between then and death.[120]

But where was the late nineteenth-century work stress epidemic? Where were the legions of counsellors? Work at the beginning of the twenty-first century may at least for some workers be more demanding than it was twenty years earlier, but even in comparison with work in the first half of the twentieth century, it can hardly be seen as the psychologically damaging, emotionally scarring, and unendurable experience portrayed in the work stress discourse.

The work stress epidemic may be a response to changes in work that have occurred since the mid-1970s, but it is broader socio-cultural changes – the heightened awareness of physical and mental vulnerability, the culture of victimhood, and the emergence of the therapeutic state – that account for experiences at work being interpreted through the medicalized prism of epidemic and disease. In the 1970s exploitation and alienation in the workplace led to strikes and the three-day week; today they lead to counselling, early retirement on medical grounds and the pursuit of financial compensation. Changes in Britain's emotional script or ethnopsychology mean that heavy workload, intensive working, coercive management and other problems at work are no longer seen as collective issues to be fought over through industrial action or political activity, but as individualized threats to the mental and physical health of the worker, to which therapeutic intervention is the proper response.

The work stress epidemic may be conditioned by socio-cultural factors outside the workplace, but it is no less 'real' for that. As the physiological evidence presented in Chapter 2 illustrates, stress has an embodied reality, in the actions of the autonomic nervous system and the hypothalamic–pituitary axis. Some of these physiological changes may even contribute to health problems such as heart disease or cancer (though the evidence here is less convincing). How can the two statements – work stress is conditioned by socio-cultural factors, and stress has a physiological reality – both be true?

To answer this question we need to return to the embodiment perspective expounded in Chapter 3. We know from the psychologists that conscious appraisal of threats and the ability to cope with them plays a fundamental role in triggering the physiological aspects of the stress response (see Chapter 2). We also know that over the life course these relationships can become written on the body, so that physiological stress responses can be triggered unconsciously without cognitive processing. Thus, people often experience stress as an autonomous response independent of their conscious will and control. The stress response is, therefore, both interpretive and unconscious. Socio-cultural factors – the ethnopsychology – have an influence on both of these dimensions as they intertwine across the life course.

In a society with a heightened awareness of physical and mental vulnerability, where mundane experiences like walking home from school without an adult chaperone or playing on an adventure playground are seen as potential causes of physical harm, and where having a working mother or sitting examinations at school are seen as a threat to mental health, children are likely to be over-socialized or over-protected. Children who are 'wrapped in cotton wool' and denied the social space in which to negotiate their own solutions to the hazards of everyday life and the difficulties of interpersonal relations are unlikely to grow up to be self-confident social agents. The external world is likely to be perceived as a threat to be avoided rather than a challenge that can be met and overcome.[121]

Throughout childhood we learn that our encounters with the external world are likely to be physically or mentally damaging – that we are likely to be victims of 'abuse', 'trauma', or 'bullying'. These perceived threats not only influence the way we think about the world, but also our physiological response to it, by embedding unconscious pathways from perception to stress response that are not mediated by cognition or consciousness.

As a result of these unconscious responses that have developed over the life course we experience problems at work as physiological symptoms. The coercive boss, the stroppy client, the time constraints, the pile of papers in the in-tray cause us to have palpitations, panic attacks, sweating, nausea, headaches, but they do this through a process that escapes us. At this point the ethnopsychology affects us in a more direct way by shaping the way in which these physiological symptoms are interpreted and invested with meaning and by providing plausible courses of action which might be taken in response. Confronted by the unpleasant symptoms of stress we are obliged to make sense of them and decide how to respond. Is that quickening of the pulse, that rush of adrenaline, anger? Is it the body preparing to fight, or is it a precursor of disease? The ethnopsychology helps us decide. 'You have a vulnerable body and mind'; 'The world is full of threats to physical and mental health, why shouldn't work be one too?'; 'The means for fighting back collectively are organizationally and ideologically defunct'; 'You are not angry or aroused, you are stressed'; 'You are a victim'; 'You need help'; 'Services are available.'

The ethnopsychology of vulnerable bodies, victimhood and the therapeutic state provides a frame of reference in which adverse experiences at work and their embodied physiological correlates can be interpreted and invested with meaning. Coupled with the therapeutic apparatus of trade union health and safety representation, occupational health services, counselling, psychotherapy and general practitioner services, the ethnopsychology also provides a mechanism for recognition and validation – a socially accepted pathway or 'career' for the work stress victim.

Earlier in this chapter we pointed out that the discursive analysis of the ethnopsychology that we were about to present was inevitably open to the criticism that it was selective and impressionistic, and that changes in discourse might not be accompanied by changes in the consciousness of individuals. The therapeutic discourse of work stress may be seductive, but what about those who resist it? We also proposed a means of addressing this methodological difficulty: by returning to the micro level of analysis and exploring the extent to which these putative cultural changes are reflected in the consciousness of individuals, specifically in relation to their beliefs and experiences regarding therapeutic interventions for work stress. It is to this analysis that we now turn.

 **5** **Therapy or resistance?**

Whatever the causes of the work stress 'epidemic', whatever it signifies about society's shifting norms and values, there is no denying its existence as one of the key problems of twenty-first-century life. We have questioned whether work stress is really an 'epidemic' in the scientific sense of the word, but there is no denying the successful claims for compensation, the early retirements on medical grounds, the consultations with general practitioners and counsellors, the numerous 'stress-busting' guides, and the widespread misery and distress that are framed within this broad and amorphous category. So how should society respond to the work stress phenomenon?

Existing responses can be divided into two groups which reflect differences in the way that the problem is conceptualized. The first approach is to locate the origins of work stress in the structure and organization of the modern workplace and to see the solution in terms of job redesign. The second approach is to locate work stress in the responses of the individual and see the solution in terms of therapeutic intervention.

Work stress and job redesign

This is the approach taken by those working in the Scandinavian tradition of work reform. As the title of Robert Karasek and Tores Theorell's book implies – *Healthy Work: Stress, Productivity and the Reconstruction of Working Life* – job redesign is seen as a panacea not just for work-related illness, but also for low productivity.[1] The authors make specific proposals for job redesign in different occupational groups, but there are seven basic criteria that distinguish a bad job from a good one.

The first criterion is *skill discretion* – in a bad job workers have no opportunity to use or develop their expertise, whereas in a good job workers are encouraged to develop and use a wide range of skills. The second criterion is *autonomy* – in bad jobs every aspect of work is monitored and regulated by a manager or a machine, whereas in a good job control over work routines is delegated to workers; they can participate in long-term planning and work at home occasionally. The third criterion is *psychological demands* – in a bad job workers face constant time pressures, or long periods of boredom, coupled with job insecurity; in a good job the demands are interspersed with learning experiences and there is greater job security. The fourth criterion is *social relations* – in a bad job workers are isolated from their colleagues and unable to build lasting supportive relations; in a good job teamworking is encouraged and new telecommunications technology is used to avoid isolation. The fifth criterion is *social rights* – in a bad job workers have few rights or responsibilities; in a good job there are democratic procedures, such as a grievance council, to protect workers from arbitrary authority. The sixth criterion is *meaningfulness/customer feedback* – in a bad job workers are detached from the needs of customers or obliged to act against the customer's interests; in a good job workers gain direct feedback from customers and work with them to produce products that adequately meet their needs. Finally, the seventh criterion is *family/work interface* – in a bad job work roles are separated from family roles leading to sex-role conflicts and family degeneration; in a good job work and family responsibilities are shared between the sexes.

The striking thing about the job redesign agenda is how much of it has nominally been achieved and how little it has contributed to the amelioration of job strain or work stress. Although Karasek and Theorell claim that their approach is applicable to the modern workplace, it really has its origins in the blue-collar manufacturing sector that prevailed for much of the twentieth century, where a predominantly male workforce was subordinated to the dull routine of the production line, repetitively performing a small number of routine tasks with little scope for developing new skills, working creatively with other workers, or obtaining direct feedback from customers. As we observed in Chapter 4, this type of work has declined rapidly over the last two decades as the service and information sectors have expanded. More women have entered the labour market, and flexibility, reskilling, teamworking and consumerism have become the buzz-words of the new economy.

Many of these developments relate very closely to Karasek and Theorell's prescription for job redesign, but ironically they have been accompanied by a rapid increase in work stress and are cited by many commentators as *causes* of the epidemic rather than a cure. Teamwork, that supposed guarantor of skill discretion, autonomy, demand control and social support, has been described by Richard Sennett as 'the group practice of demeaning superficiality'.[2] Rather than giving workers an enhanced sense of 'meaning-fulness' or 'personal pride', the growth of consumerism coupled with Total Quality Management and the banalities of 'Have a Nice Day' customer relations has become another stick for managers to beat them with. Tele-communications technology, such as the mobile phone, laptop computer and e-mail, may have reduced isolation but it has also extended the scope of managerial surveillance and produced 'information overload'. It seems that yesterday's cures for work stress are today's causes.

The difficulty is that the job redesign agenda is posited as a top-down technical/managerial fix within the existing structure of economic relations. The defining characteristic of wage labour is that workers exchange their labour power for a wage and in so doing lose the right to control their pro-ductive activity. Within the boundaries of this exchange there is considerable scope for variation in the way in which work is organized and the extent to which workers' interests are prioritized (the difference between Karasek and Theorell's 'good' and 'bad' jobs), but the relationship remains a funda-mentally antagonistic one. Private companies must return a profit, the public sector must provide services within tight budgets. Under these circumstances new technologies and methods of working which might otherwise reduce the drudgery and enhance the experience of work often become ways of reinforcing the worker's alienation. This does not mean that significant con-cessions cannot be granted, but it seems unlikely that they will be introduced by management without significant pressure from workers, and, as we saw in Chapter 4, the means by which such pressure has traditionally been applied (through militant trade unionism) are no longer effective.

The widespread belief that there is no alternative to the managerial logic of late capitalism has led to a new fatalism and a rejection of the optimistic claims of the job redesign and workers' democracy movement. The claim that work can be re-engineered at the macro level to achieve the twin goals of a happy workforce and raised productivity appears naïve in the age of the call centre, and the grand project of job redesign has been replaced by a narrower focus on the minutiae of working life, exemplified by the modest goals of the 'time management course', and the 'team-building exercise'. The new mantra is 'Don't work harder; work smarter', and it implies a shift from a collective workforce perspective towards individualized coping techniques and efficient working practices.

As we saw in Chapter 1, the macro policy agenda for work reform has not been entirely abandoned; New Labour in party with the European Union has introduced a series of reforms governing the minimum wage, the length of the working week, work–life balance etc. However, quite apart from their modest scope, the real significance of such measures lies in their assump-tions about the nature of work and human potential. In the 1960s and 1970s the Scandinavian work reform movement was based on the optimistic assumption that a wholesale reorganization of the workplace would not only lead to greater happiness and fulfilment among workers, it would also unleash the human potential for creativity, innovation and productivity – it was about achieving more, not less. The new agenda for work reform is based on far more pessimistic assumptions, not just about the scope for transforming the workplace, but also concerning human potential and resilience. On one hand, the structure and organization of the workplace is perceived to be largely the product of global economic forces that are independent from political will. The contemporary mode of work is viewed as an unstoppable Leviathan, to be guarded against rather than fundamentally transformed. On the other hand, it is also assumed that the human potential for resilience, endurance and achievement is close to being exhausted by the demands of paid employment. It is as if there is a 'natural' limit to what humans can achieve or endure, dictated by biological constraints on the body and mind. The imaginary within which government policy on work is framed is that of the 'unstoppable force' of modern production colliding with the 'immoveable object' of human endurance. The objective is no longer to transform work, but simply to make it survivable by chipping away at the length of the working week, outlawing 'starvation' wages, implementing a minimal right to paternity leave.

Such reforms, modest as they are, may be welcome, but they are widely seen as a means of limiting the 'damage' of the contemporary mode of work, rather than as a serious challenge to it. The contradiction becomes apparent when we consider the Labour government's plans to improve public services by increasing the role of the private sector, and the character of the trade union response to these proposals.[3] Involving the private sector is seen as the *only* way of addressing the inefficiency and inertia of institutions like the National Health Service. The importation of private sector working practices, organizational mechanisms, managerial techniques and funding arrangements is considered to have an immutable logic. The Prime Minister backed up this claim by describing a project in Glasgow which saw 29 schools built or renovated in three years with private sector help – 'Left to the public sector, the project would take 25 years.' However, 'modernization' of this kind is also perceived to come at a high cost for the workforce. The assumption is that the reforms will push an already hard-pressed workforce beyond the limit of what can be endured. Thus, the trade union response has focused on the effects that the reforms will have on the morale of NHS workers. The logic of the free market is not contested, only its consequences for the well-being of the workforce. The matter will doubtless be resolved when the proposals for private involvement are matched by measures to safeguard the interests of the employees. In this sense the government's macro policies on work are couched within a therapeutic idiom rather than a political one. This leads into the second, and, we would argue, dominant response to the work stress phenomenon; treating it as an individual problem that requires therapeutic intervention.

Work stress and therapy

Although the job redesign agenda can still be found in the academic discourse on work stress, the public discourse is overwhelmingly concerned with various forms of therapy. The various 'therapies' available for work stress vary in terms of their formality. At the informal end of the spectrum there is a vast range of 'stress-busting' guides, stress management and relaxation techniques that can be found in popular magazines, books and short courses. Moreover, many leisure, exercise and personal care activities (such as massage and yoga) are marketed as ways of combating stress. Most of these are offered without any reference to empirical evidence of their efficacy and their main claim is often that they offer a means of achieving relaxation which is seen as the opposite of stress.

Further along the continuum are the various alternative or complementary therapies, such as acupuncture, chiropractic, homeopathy, aromatherapy and reflexology which, though not exclusively concerned with stress, do claim to reorder the body physically in ways which will either remove the negative physical consequences of stress or offer greater resilience. Again, the evidence base for such interventions is usually far from conclusive and legitimacy is sought by reference to a non-biomedical cosmology. Alongside the established alternative therapies there are a range of other physiological interventions that are solely concerned with treating or managing stress. Biofeedback, for instance, in which physiological indicators such as blood pressure or body temperature are constantly measured and the results fed back to the 'patient' who then learns to reduce them by relaxing. Stress-dots are perhaps the most simplistic form of biofeedback.[4] They comprise a small plastic dot that is stuck on to the skin, usually on the back of the hand, which is made from a heat-sensitive material (the same as that used in fish-tank thermometers). It is claimed that as an individual is exposed to stress, skin temperature will increase and the dot will change colour, indicating the need to calm down and relax (although presumably the same effect could be achieved by standing next to a radiator).

Psychotherapeutic techniques such as counselling and cognitive behaviour modification cross the boundary between informal and formal care as they are often available privately (sometimes through an employer) or through general practice. The most that can be said of the evidence base for such interventions is that it is contested.[5] Despite this, counselling in particular has become widely available, with over 50 per cent of British general practices offering the service.[6] General practitioners have a range of other treatment options available to them including medication, referral to a psychiatrist, or simply the granting of sick leave.

Many of the therapies for work stress are organized around the principle of arousal avoidance or arousal containment. The assumption is that relaxation is a healthier emotional state than arousal and that controlling the physiological processes of arousal throughout a stressful experience, for example by practising muscle relaxing techniques at work, or by returning to a relaxed state soon afterwards, will effectively counter any adverse psychological or physical health problems that might otherwise result. Angela Patmore has suggested that this assumption amounts to the pursuit of a 'tranquillized society' where stimulating and exciting experiences are pathologized.[7] Moreover, the arousal avoidance perspective overlooks the adaptive value of the stress response, i.e. its value as a means of preparing the body for action. Patmore refers to the way in which athletes and performance artists manipulate the stress response – 'psyching' themselves up in order to boost or enrich their performance. Arousal avoidance amounts to a lowering of expectations about what can be achieved; it is a form of retreat from demanding and challenging experiences and the sense of exhilaration and achievement that comes from meeting them. Although, in their defence, the advocates of stress management might argue that increasing arousal only adds to performance up to a certain point after which the graph flattens and then dips, and that their techniques aim to enable people to stay at the top of the curve.

Whatever the consequences such therapies have for individual resilience (a theme we return to later in the chapter), there remain a series of questions about the political consequences of addressing the problem of work stress through a therapeutic idiom. Does this amount to an individualization of what is essentially a social and economic problem? Does it extend the power of the medical profession? Is it about governance, i.e. regulating behaviour and defusing dissent? These questions about the scope and deployment of medical power have exercised sociologists for a generation, and there is value in considering this literature.

The medicalization thesis

The medicalization thesis emerged in the late 1960s and early 1970s as part of a broader critique of prevailing social relations, institutional arrangements and bodies of social knowledge. It concerns the extent to which behaviours and problems which were previously not thought of as medical issues, for example alcohol consumption and diet, have been brought under medical jurisdiction.[8–9] Many writers have explored this issue and there are differences in emphasis and interpretation. In his critique Strong lists ten key propositions of the medicalization thesis; however, they can be condensed into three closely interrelated key themes: the extension of professional power, social control, and a critique of the biomedical model. Thus for Eliot Friedson, medicalization is fundamentally about medical dominance, and the conscious pursuit of a strategy on the part of the medical profession to define and control health and illness.[10] Not only does this entail broadening the range of problems defined as medical, but also driving out non-medical practitioners, or at least subordinating them to professional control; for example, Ann Oakley has analysed the way in which child-birth was transformed from a 'natural' process supervised by lay midwives into a technological issue governed by the predominantly male medical profession.[11-12]

This leads into the second dimension of the medicalization thesis: the process of social control, not just of subordinate occupational groups, but also of patients and the wider population. We partially explored this issue in Chapter 3 in relation to the rise of the therapeutic state. The feminist critique of the way in which women's bodies are increasingly subjected to control by a patriarchal medical profession is also relevant here.[13-14] Others have described the way in which medical knowledge has been used in the regulation and control of madness.[15-16] The doctor's state sanctioned control over medical knowledge and resources, coupled with the right to validate sickness claims (and, in the instance of mental illness, mobilize the coercive powers of the state), amounts to a massive imbalance of power between the professional and patient.

Medicine may be implicated in the exercise of social control, but is this primarily in the interests of the medical profession as Friedson suggests? Other beneficiaries have also been suggested, including the capitalist class,[17] the pharmaceutical industry, and lay pressure groups representing deviants.[18] As well as facilitating direct control over patients' lives, medicalization also depoliticizes social problems, by advocating individualized interventions rather than socio-economic solutions, a by-product of which is the patient's dependence upon professionals.

The third key theme of the medicalization thesis concerns the status of the biomedical model and the scientific knowledge based upon it. Mishler has cited four characteristics of the biomedical model: disease as deviation from normal biological functioning; the doctrine of specific aetiology; the generic nature of disease; and the claim that medical knowledge is value-free.[19] As well as taking issue with the biological reductionism of the model, critics have also questioned the positivist assumptions on which it is putat-ively based, and which gives the impression of a linear progression from superstition to enlightenment:

> The concrete record of scientific and medical development assumes without question that there are solid facts to discover and that the con-tinuous discovery of these facts leads eventually to the state of know-ledge we have today. But this very assumption automatically isolates the endeavour called 'scientific' or 'medical' advancement from its social context. That is, it neither examines the non-intellectual contingencies which mould ideas, nor does it look at the use of scientific or medical concepts as cultural, social, religious or ideological tools.[20]

It is the scientificity of the biomedical model, coupled with the fact that it cannot be easily systematized and routinized,[21] that underpins the process of medicalization, legitimating the extensive powers of the medical profession, the relative powerlessness of the patient, and the marginalization of non-medical practitioners and policies. Ivan Illich rehearses the key themes of the medicalization thesis in his book *Medical Nemesis*, the main claim of which is that modern medicine does more harm than good. He cites three types of 'iatrogenesis': *clinical* (physical harm caused by medical intervention); *social* (seeing medical care as the solution to all our ills); and *structural* (the destruction of patient autonomy and responsibility).[22] This assault on the achievements of modern medicine is often reinforced by reference to the claim that the remarkable improvements in health and longevity that have occurred since the nineteenth century owe more to rising living standards and public health measures than they do to high-technology medicine.[23]

As it stood in the early 1980s the medicalization thesis seems very relevant to our account of the work stress phenomenon. The discourse of work stress does appear to reduce what might previously have been considered to be the political and economic issues of adverse experiences at work to the individualized domain of therapeutic practice, extending the scope of the medical model (and the regulatory powers of the medical profession) into yet another sphere of everyday life. Similarly, the body of 'scientific knowledge' on which the discourse is based can be criticized for its naturalizing and universalizing positivism.[24] Moreover, as we will argue below, seeking medical care for the problem of work stress may have adverse consequences for the 'patient' in terms of self-identity and future career. However, following the radical and sometimes sweeping claims of the 1970s the medicalization thesis was subjected to extensive criticism and revision which will be examined before considering its relevance to the work stress phenomenon.

The point of departure for reviewing the medicalization thesis is Strong's 1979 paper on 'sociological imperialism', recently revisited by Williams.[25–6] Strong's argument claims that the sociological critique of medical power is not only a gross distortion, but one which is self-serving, because it attempts to displace the biomedical model with the counter-claims of the 'social model' of health and illness, which amounts to imperialist rivalry. Strong's critique covers the three central claims of the medicalization thesis discussed above.

First, regarding the expansion of medical power, Strong argues that the analysis is historically naïve, for example in claiming that childbirth was free from the exercise of power and control prior to the ascendance of the medical profession – domination was still exercised, but with less satisfactory results. Similarly, rather than a homogeneous group ruthlessly pursuing a uniform professional agenda, Strong sees a more diverse network of subdisciplines which are not 'all of one mind'. Nor does the profession have an unquenchable appetite for expanding its sphere of influence, pragmatically retreating from or 'demedicalizing' areas where medicine has little to offer, and limiting entry to the profession. Moreover, the state plays an important role in limiting medical expansion (not least by the imposition of financial constraints), and safeguarding 'bourgeois freedoms'.

Secondly, Strong suggests that the medicalization thesis distorts the extent to which medical practice is implicated in social control. Doctors may decide which treatments to offer, but patients usually (though not always) retain the right to decline them. Similarly, the patient's alleged dependence on clinical intervention is overstated. More recent evidence suggests that many doctors are at least ambivalent if not decidedly reluctant to exercise what they see as moral regulation of their patients' life choices.[27-8]

Thirdly, and perhaps most convincingly, Strong argues that the critique of the biomedical model and the knowledge based upon it is highly selective and misleading. Others have observed that the caricature of the medical model presented in many accounts of the medicalization thesis which emphasizes simple cause and effect relationships and biological reductionism are rarely found in contemporary practice, which tends to adopt a more holistic approach.[29] Moreover, the historical balance sheet of the costs and benefits of medical practice is distorted by the advocates of medicalization who tend to exaggerate the disasters and false starts and understate the triumphs.

In short, while Strong recognizes the need for critical scrutiny of professional power,[30] the claims of the medicalization thesis overstate the extent to which it is implicated in social control and underestimate the genuine contribution it has made to the amelioration of human illness and pain, as Williams concludes:

> When we are ill, when the uncertainties and contingencies of our mortal bodies and their fleshy demise are all too apparent, recourse to medicine may seem an eminently preferable option to the relativising spirit and deconstructive desires of postmodernism.[31]

From a post-millennial vantage point the critique of professional power takes on an almost Thatcherite gloss, and commentators have become more concerned with the extent to which clinicians are increasingly subordinated to managerial surveillance and regulation than with their attempts to expand their power and status. The challenge to medical autonomy and power has not just come from government, but also from a more questioning (and litigious)[32] population, the rise of alternative therapies,[33] and the professionalization of other occupational groups, particularly nurses.[34] Whether these challenges mark a fundamental shift in the balance of power or simply an uncomfortable period of readjustment remains to be seen.[35-6]

The claim that the power of the medical profession might be waning rather than waxing has a history as long as the medicalization thesis.[37-8]

As well as puncturing the myth of the omnipotent doctor critics have also challenged the assumption that the patient is simply the passive subject of medicalization:

> The lay public are not simply passive and dependent upon modern medicine, nor are they necessarily duped by medical ideology and technology. Rather many forms of 'counter reaction' are beginning to emerge; responses that challenge any simple portrayal of the modern individual as passive in the face of modern medicine. Seen in this light, the notion of a 'blanket dependence' on medicine or the fabrication of 'docile bodies' appears to have a somewhat hollow ring to it, resulting in a largely 'overdrawn' view of medical power, dominance and control.[39]

The emergence of the 'active patient' contesting professional wisdom and decision making does not always result in a rejection of medicalization. Indeed, patients may actively pursue clinical recognition and validation of their problems as 'authentic' pathology to bolster their claims-making behaviour, even where medical opinion is equivocal or sceptical, for example in relation to new 'diseases' such as repetitive strain injury,[40] chronic fatigue syndrome[41] and Gulf war syndrome.[42] This putative renegotiation of the traditional doctor–patient relationship, characterized by ambivalence about professional expertise and integrity and a reassertion of the validity of lay experience, should be placed in the context of broader social changes that characterize 'late modernity'.

In Chapter 4 we described the heightened sense of physical and mental vulnerability that is characterized by the large number of health scares and panics that have occurred since the early 1990s. However, this has not been accompanied by unequivocal support for the 'technical fix'. In earlier times natural phenomena were seen as the main risks to human health and well-being, with technical and scientific knowledge viewed as the source of solutions. In late modernity human intervention in nature is viewed with greater ambivalence, with scientific knowledge and expert systems increasingly viewed as a potential risk as well as a remedy.[43–4] The age of uncritical trust in the experts, if it ever existed, is now gone, replaced by a desire to reappropriate knowledge and skills that were previously reserved for professionals, a process which Giddens refers to as lay reskilling.[45]

Since its emergence at the beginning of the 1970s the criticisms of the medicalization thesis have mounted; from Strong's account of its many distortions and exaggerations, through the many challenges to the power and autonomy of the medical profession, up to the emergence of demedicalization and lay reskilling. What then, if anything, can be salvaged from the wreckage? First, it is important to note a category error that can be found among critics of medicalization as well as among some of its supporters: the conflation of the intentional pursuit of power and influence on the part of the medical profession with a broader tendency to explain experiences within a medicalized idiom.[46] The two are not mutually exclusive – the Royal Colleges and other professional bodies may in the past have consciously sought to extend the range of medical jurisdiction in the interests of their members – but any setbacks or limitations on the autonomy and power of the medical profession do not automatically amount to a diminution of society's therapeutic imperative. The so-called 'social model' posited as an alternative to biomedicine has, as Strong prophesied, simply extended the medical gaze into new areas of everyday life,[47] even if some medical practitioners are uneasy about this intrusion. Similarly, accounts of lay reskilling, consumerism, self-help and support groups[48] do not so much represent a retreat from the medical model as a broadening of its 'personnel' to include non-professionals and patients.

This leads into a further refinement of the medicalization thesis which differentiates between three different levels of medicalization – conceptual, institutional and doctor–patient interaction.[49] Renegotiating the terms of the doctor–patient relationship and stepping outside the formal institutions of the medical apparatus do not necessarily entail a radical departure from the conceptual framework of medical/therapeutic discourse. It is, for instance, possible to adopt the self-identity of the work stress victim, to interpret adverse experiences at work through the medicalized categories of pathology, to seek therapeutic support and treatment, without once engaging with formal health care institutions or the doctor–patient relationship. It is this capacity for discourse to provide an explanatory framework through which experiences can be interpreted and invested with meaning, and to constitute particular forms of subjectivity, that is the most abiding legacy of the medicalization thesis. This shift of focus away from the self-interested strategies of the medical profession towards the role of medical discourse in constituting self-identity leads inevitably into consideration of the work of Michel Foucault.

Although Foucault might have bridled at such a Whiggish proposition, there is a clear line of development in his treatment of power and knowledge. In his early work – *Madness and Civilisation*,[50] *Discipline and Punish*,[51] *The Birth of the Clinic*[52] – Foucault was concerned with the historical development of regimens of knowledge and their implication in the exercise of social control. Power was conceptualized as an external force acting on the individual who was a passive object of surveillance and regulation – a 'docile body'. As Lupton has observed,[53] these early formulations emerged at the same time as the medicalization thesis and there are many parallels between the two approaches, not least the notion of a passive subject subordinated to powerful disciplines.

However, later in his career Foucault became less interested in domination by external agencies and shifted his attention to the ways in which we formulate our own subjectivity within the constraints and incitements of discourse, using what he described as 'technologies of the self':

Perhaps I've insisted too much on the technology of domination and power. I am more interested in the interaction between oneself and others and in the technologies of individual domination, the history of how an individual acts upon himself, in the technology of the self.[54]

Thus, in *The History of Sexuality*[55] Foucault examines the way in which the discourse on sexuality gives rise to new subjectivities and identities – the hysterical woman, the masturbating child, the homosexual. These identities were not simply imposed by external agents of domination, but internalized by the subject as a means of making sense of his experiences, for example, homosexuality stopped being something you *do* and became something you *are*. These issues of the formation of the self are explored at greater length in Chapter 3. The important point here is the extent to which Foucault's later work betrays a fundamental shift in his conception of power. He no longer sees the exercise of power as purely repressive and imposed by external agents of domination, but as a positive creative force which incites new behaviours, identities and modes of being, and which is adopted by the subject rather than imposed from above.

This reconceptualization of the micro-relations of power marks a radical departure from earlier formulations of the medicalization thesis. The patient–doctor relationship is no longer one in which a passive subject or 'docile body' is subordinated by a 'figure of domination'; the doctor is simply a nodal point through which power passes and the patient is an active participant in the exercise of power.[56–7] Medical discourse becomes something which is actively appropriated and used, or contested and rejected, by the patient. It is the dialectical and phenomenological character of this process that provides the basis for resistance. However, within the Foucauldian perspective the emancipatory potential of resistance is limited by epistemological constraints. Foucault claimed that he was not interested in the distinction between truth and falsity so much as the way in which effects of truth were achieved. Some of his followers have adopted an even more overt relativism in relation to medical knowledge:

A body analysed for humours contains humours; a body analysed for organs and tissues is constituted by organs and tissues; a body analysed for psychosocial functioning is a psychosocial object.[58]

Such relativism is a luxury that can only be enjoyed by the healthy. Galen and William Harvey both theorized the circulation of the blood – Harvey was right, Galen was wrong. Surgery based on the Galenic system would likely result in the patient's death, that based on Harvey's theory can save lives and ameliorate suffering.[59] Medical knowledge may be a product of its time and place; it may be open to distortion, manipulation, false claims; it may be used to oppress, control, pacify and offend against the patient's interests in a multitude of ways, but the material reality of the body pro-vides a means of testing such truth claims. It is this materiality and the demonstrable benefits of many clinical interventions that makes biomed-icine such a compelling discursive formation. The large number of clinical successes (compared with the small number of disasters like thalidomide) is a powerful source of legitimation even where the evidence and observable benefits are less convincing, for instance in health promotion or therapies for work stress.

The difficulty arises because the material reality of the body is not access-ible in an unmediated form. We rely on discourse as an aid to making sense of the signs and symptoms of the body – what Shilling refers to as the phenomenology of the body.[60] In choosing how to act, what to accept or reject, we oscillate between our lived experience of the body and various interpretive frameworks – medical science, lay epidemiology, alternative medicine, folk beliefs and superstitions. Moreover, although evidence of clinical effectiveness is compelling, there are other, non-medical, costs and benefits to be weighed. Adopting a 'healthy lifestyle' may (or may not) reduce morbidity and extend longevity in the future, but in the short term it entails foregoing the pleasures of tobacco and alcohol and enduring the discipline of diet and exercise regimens. Rather than a passive object of medical domination, the patient is a conscious subject, appraising the claims of biomedicine, negotiating the terms of clinical intervention, exploring alternative strategies and predicting outcomes.

The relativist dismissal of biomedicine (and scientific knowledge generally) as simply another socially constructed cultural product that offers no better grasp of reality than unaided common sense is even more unsatisfactory than the counter-view that science simply reports objective facts about reality unmediated by social or cultural influences. The former view is profoundly pessimistic and anti-humanist; it assumes that rational thought and the con-trol afforded by the experimental method offers no advance over superstition and prejudice. Fortunately, as Kenan Malik has observed, we need not settle for either view:

> Science certainly gives us access to a reality that exists independently of human beings. In this sense science is different from other forms of knowledge, such as politics or literature. But the scientific process does not stand apart from the culture it inhabits. The questions scientists ask about the world, and the interpretations they place on their data, are often shaped by cultural attitudes, needs and possibilities. In most scientific disciplines, the cultural context does not impress too deeply upon the scientific answers.[61]

Malik goes on to cite Nobel Prize-winning physicist Steven Weinberg's observation that in most cases the cultural influences on scientific discoveries get 'refined away, like slag from ore'.[62] Scientific methods of 'refinement' enable us to make reliable predictions and exercise a high degree of control over the unconscious objects of the material world, but as we observed in Chapters 2 and 3, these strategies quickly break down when it comes to studying the conscious meaningful behaviour of sentient human beings, where subjective emotional states, motivations and interpretations hold sway. The problem with biomedical knowledge is that it spans the duality of the human body as an object and a subject. It can make objective statements about the body, for instance, concerning the circulation and composition of the blood, the functioning of organs, the physiological effects of administering different compounds or substances. This is vital knowledge of immense value to the patient and explains why despite occasional blunders biomedical knowledge and clinical expertise are held in such high regard. However, this objective knowledge of the body is bound up with the subjective process of making sense of the world and choosing how to act. And it is here that the cultural and social factors re-enter clinical practice through the assumptions that are made about 'human nature' and the foreclosing of alternative strategies.

Take the issue of tobacco smoking and lung cancer. The existence of epidemiological evidence of an association between the two can hardly be described as an act of oppression. However, the moral imperative to stop smoking, the creation of a negative identity for smokers (as feckless and irresponsible), the construction of 'explanations' of smoking behaviour (physical addiction, information deficit, peer group pressure, low self-esteem, response to stress or poverty), the development of 'appropriate' smoking cessation strategies (information provision, nicotine patches, counselling, community empowerment in deprived areas), the adoption of coercive policies on taxation of tobacco and banning smoking in public places, go far beyond scientific analysis of the material body. They amount to a colonization of the lifeworld based on cultural assumptions about human values and historically specific claims about which choices are viable or desirable. It is in this apparently seamless transition from the objective world of science to the subjective world of conscious agency that the antagonism and ambivalence of the doctor–patient relationship resides. As a nodal point for bio-power the doctor is simultaneously both redeemer and oppressor; the source of literally life-saving knowledge and resources, but also the transmitter of agency-robbing identities and strategies which may limit personal autonomy.

If the science did not work this transition would be more difficult to sustain. However, although the science or treatment often does work, at least within the terms of its own frame of reference, the end result of the medicalization process – the adoption of a new subjectivity or self-identity – is not a foregone conclusion. Active resistance always remains a possibility. Bloor and MacIntosh conducted a qualitative study of Scottish mothers receiving home visits from health visitors. Rather than surrendering to medical power and having their behaviour shaped by surveillance and regulation, many of the mothers resisted in various ways, by concealing information, telling lies, refusing to cooperate, or challenging the value and legitimacy of the health visitor's advice.[63] From her own research into the doctor–patient relationship Lupton concludes:

> When consulting a doctor, individuals may, on at least some occasions, and if they so choose, attempt to struggle against, challenge or subvert those disciplinary techniques they experience as restricting their autonomy. That patients often fail to take 'doctor's orders' is evident in the extensive literature on the problem of patient compliance with medical regimens. On the other hand, those individuals who 'go along' with medical advice need not be viewed as passively accepting the orders of the medical gaze, but rather could be seen as engaging in practices of the self that they consider are vital to their own well being and freedom from discomfort or pain.[64]

Our analysis has brought us some way from the initial formulations of the medicalization thesis with their emphasis on the conscious pursuit of power by the medical profession, the domination and control of the passive unresisting patient, and the dismissal of biomedicine as iatrogenic and ideological. The criticisms and reformulations of the original thesis point to a far more nuanced and dialectical model which continues the theme of social control without the need for a conspiracy theory of professional imperialism, or the wholesale rejection of medical knowledge, or seeing the patient as a passive stooge. The medical model may lure us into adopting agency-robbing subjectivities with the promise of scientific solutions to our problems, but we are by no means powerless in the face of these incitements to infirmity. Rather, it seems our relationship to the therapeutic apparatus is one of reflexive negotiation, in which resistance may figure just as prominently as compliance.

In earlier chapters we have charted the scientific, cultural, economic and political factors that have given rise to the work stress discourse and to the social identity of the work stress victim. We have argued that these factors also push the work stress victim towards a therapeutic solution. Yet not all (or even most) of the people who define their problems through the medicalized discourse of work stress seek clinical intervention. Why in the face of such persuasive incitements do so many choose to resist? What are the factors that influence help-seeking behaviour? What happens to those who do seek a therapeutic solution? Are their symptoms ameliorated by the available treatments? And what consequences does the receipt of therapy have for their self-identity, future resilience and career? To address these questions we return to empirical evidence from our own research.

Lay perspectives on therapy and resistance

The following data come from the Dover study, some of the findings of which were presented in Chapter 1. A two-stage design was adopted: a community postal questionnaire survey (to which 1385 people responded) followed up by qualitative interviews with a subsample of 20 informants. A detailed account of the methodology is given in the Appendix.

In the survey respondents were asked if they had ever sought advice from their doctor, or another health professional, about coping with depression or anxiety caused by work stress; 14 per cent of workers reported that they had. The questionnaire listed different potential sources of help and all respondents (not just those in work) were asked to indicate which, if any, they had consulted regarding stress, anxiety and depression (not specifically work-related) during the previous 12 months. Informal support from family and friends was the most popular source of help (35 per cent), followed by the family doctor (24 per cent). Only 5 per cent of respondents reported that they had consulted a counsellor. Of those in work, 13 per cent had consulted a manager. All other sources of help had consultation rates below 5 per cent.

A similar question was asked of all respondents about whom they would seek help from if they were to suffer anxiety or depression in the future. Over 70 per cent reported that they would consult their doctor, 68 per cent would go to family and friends and less than 20 per cent would seek help from a counsellor.

Of those that had already consulted their family doctor about stress or depression nearly 50 per cent had been prescribed medication, 46 per cent had been asked to come again if their symptoms did not improve, 20 per cent had been issued with a sick note, 15 per cent had been referred to a counsellor or psychotherapist and 8 per cent had been referred to a psychiatrist or community psychiatric nurse.

In themselves these figures tell us little about the work stress 'epidemic' and there are clearly difficulties in generalizing from a small study in a particular locality. However, the quantitative data do provide a useful backdrop for the findings of the follow-up interviews. That 14 per cent of workers had consulted their family doctor specifically about work stress suggests that problems at work are being 'medicalized' by a substantial proportion of the workforce. However, informal support from family and friends still appears to be the favoured means of addressing anxiety and depression. Similarly, despite the wide availability of counselling services and the high public profile of counselling, many people appear to be reluctant to use it. A significant proportion of patients had been referred to psychotherapeutic and psychiatric services by their GP, but medication was a more frequent course of action.

This section is concerned with what happens when people seek medical advice about problems attributed to work stress. What influences their decision to consult? What treatment do they receive, and are they satisfied with what they get? What role does the clinician play in defining the cause of their problems? Do such people become dependent on their clinician or counsellor? What impact does consultation have on their lives, particularly those who take early retirement on medical grounds? Of course, not everyone who experiences symptoms that they associate with work stress decides to consult a clinician. So before addressing the above questions it is important to examine alternative strategies for managing work stress, and the factors that influence the decision to consult.

The problem with quantitative data is that they tell us nothing of the reasoning behind people's choices or the way they interpret or give meaning to their experiences. In order to access this subjective data follow-up interviews were conducted with informants who had scored highly on quantitative measures of job strain, such as high job demands, lack of control over work and lack of support from colleagues and managers. The informants were mixed in terms of their reported levels of mental distress and whether or not they had consulted a doctor about their work-related problems. We began by asking informants to describe what work stress meant to them and the effects they felt it had on them. These data are reported in Chapter 1. Following on from this we asked informants how they dealt with the problems they defined as work stress.

Informal methods of managing work stress

When asked how they went about dealing with stress, many informants mentioned a range of behaviours which might be described as negative or potentially health damaging, for instance smoking, heavy drinking, kicking or throwing things, and 'blowing your top' either at work or at home. Other strategies were more positive, for instance using humour to defuse stress at work or taking informal breaks to get away from a stressful situation. Outside work, supportive conversations with family and friends were often felt to be an effective way of unwinding from the pressures of work. Other informants reported using alternative therapies such as aromatherapy, massage, and relaxation techniques, although their efficacy was often perceived to be limited:

> I pay somebody to do me a massage. That's every three weeks. I go to a place at Faversham where you can have a jacuzzi, sauna, massage and a day there.

> *Do those sort of things help with the work stress?*

> Not in the slightest. I don't relax under a massage anyway. No I don't find that relaxing. You know, they say you should play all this soppy music, lay on the floor and think of your feet, and then your knees, and it just doesn't do anything for me.

Not all informants were as dismissive of the alternative therapies, but they tended to be reported as effective only where the informant was experiencing fairly minor stress-related symptoms. Where symptoms had become more severe, it was often suggested that such techniques were no longer effective. It was often at this point that medical advice was sought.

Deciding whether to consult

Severity of symptoms was the most common reason for consultation among informants who had sought help from their doctor. Those who had not consulted were asked under what circumstances they would be willing to. Many suggested that they would only be willing to consult if they experienced symptoms that were severe enough to affect their work or other aspects of their life:

> *Under what sort of circumstances do you think you would be willing to go to your doctor* [with problems arising from work stress]?
>
> I think if it was making me very ill and I wasn't able to do my job properly or live my life as well, because I think if it's going to disrupt your life that much, then obviously something has got to be done about it.

Many informants expressed a reluctance to visit their doctor with problems they associated with work stress, even where 'symptoms' were quite severe. There seemed to be a widespread awareness that seeking professional help for an emotional or psychological problem would entail crossing an often unspecified boundary which they were reluctant to do without the encouragement of others. Some had only attended after being urged to do so by colleagues:

> I was working on the ship and I was just feeling quite tearful and one of the girls said to me, 'You go to the doctors and get signed off.'

Even where symptoms were very pronounced and informants had felt obliged to visit their doctor, there was still often a reluctance to enter fully into a therapeutic regimen. In some instances visiting the doctor was seen simply as a means of legitimating absence from work:

> The doctor was just a means to an end to get a sick note because I wasn't fit enough to work. I didn't feel that the doctor herself actually talked to me and helped me, no. At that time I couldn't continue work.

Even where a visit to the doctor was simply to obtain sick leave, there was often an awareness that this still involved a degree of medicalization. The doctor can grant absence from work, but only by defining problems at work in terms of their consequences for physical, or more frequently mental, health. Formally entering the sick role in this way was often perceived to be stigmatizing and a potential source of future problems, for instance several informants were reluctant to consult their GP because they were worried that references to work stress and mental health problems in their medical records might adversely affect their future job prospects:

> . . . if you are put off sick with anxiety and depression [. . .] and it goes on for any length of time, it's certainly going to affect your work prospects. So you're very wary about having that put on your medical record; that you suffer from any mental illness.

Concerns about the hidden 'costs' of consulting the doctor were matched by scepticism about the likely benefits of attendance, particularly concerning psychological problems. Not only were some informants reluctant to 'waste the doctor's time', there was also a widely held belief that consultation would only result in a prescription for medication, which was not only unlikely to resolve the underlying causes of work stress, but might also have adverse consequences:

> You generally put it to the back of your mind and carry on and keep going, that's the only way to cope with it. If the headaches get a bit too much you can have a little trip to the doctor's, but that doesn't usually do you any good. He takes your blood pressure, that's fine, so it's 'stress' and that's the end of the story. One time they offered me tablets, but I declined. That is a personal thing; my sister started on those and turned out to be a drug addict. I'm anti anti-depressants and that sort of thing anyway, and after all it is not solving the problem; you still wake up the next morning and it's still there. You've just got to cope with it.

The scepticism expressed by some informants about the potential benefits of clinical consultation reinforces the criticisms and limitations of the early formulations of the medicalization thesis advanced above. How can it be argued that the discourse of work stress entails a shift from a political or economic conceptualization of problems at work, towards a medicalized conception, if many informants were reluctant to consult their doctor about work stress because they doubted the efficacy of clinical intervention? The evidence is far more consistent with later conceptions of medicalization where the patient is viewed as an active questioning subject rather than the passive object of medical domination.

Scepticism about the potential efficacy of clinical intervention does not necessarily mean that a biomedical model of work stress has been replaced by a focus on tackling the structural and organizational causes of problems at work. Many of those who were reluctant to consult their doctor felt the way they did not because they did not conceptualize their problems in terms of mental health or the medical model, but because they felt that they should be able to cope with those problems by themselves, without clinical intervention:

How did you feel about going to the doctor with that kind of problem?

Pathetic, basically. You should be able to cope with life, shouldn't you; be stronger willed and get on with everything?

We reported in Chapter 1 that informants tended to conceptualize the link between problems at work and symptoms of ill health in terms of a reserve of well-being that was slowly depleted by problems at work and other external factors, and that when the reserve was exhausted ill health would follow. However, the comments about 'coping' suggest that this process was not viewed as unconscious or automatic, but as something that could be (or even *should* be) struggled against:

> ... nurses feel that they have to cope because they're the strong ones, and not have these problems, and that you can handle them yourself without outside intervention. You know about relaxation, and I should be able to manage myself without any kind of intervention.

This does not amount to a rejection of the medicalized category of work stress because the appropriate domain for action is still perceived to be the individual who must manage his or her own mental health. However, definition of the problem within a medical frame of reference does not necessarily entail passive acceptance of a therapeutic regimen, nor does it automatically include an uncontested acceptance of the patient identity. Changes in the ethnopsychology, described in Chapter 4, may have diminished people's resilience and acted as an 'incitement to infirmity', but evidence from this study suggests that many people are still reluctant to accept the social identity of someone who is unable to cope with life's demands without therapeutic input. A high value is placed on the ability to cope without professional intervention, partly because of doubts about the effectiveness of 'treatments', partly because of concerns about future employment prospects, but also because failure to cope was often perceived as a sign of weakness. Not only was this seen as stigmatizing, i.e. adversely affecting how an individual was perceived by others, but also as damaging to the individual's self-image. For instance one informant who had received medical care felt that she was unable to discuss her experiences with anyone but her closest relatives and friends:

> ... you feel you're letting yourself down because you haven't been able to cope. You feel that you have an image that you have to maintain. I've told a few close friends and the rest you tend not to talk to about it.

Although the category of work stress entails a medicalization of problems at work, there remains a strong moral imperative against formally entering the sick role and receiving medical care. Although some of the informants had quite severe symptoms, they were still reluctant to consult their doctor, not just because they were concerned about the efficacy of the treatment they would receive, but because they recognized that to do so would entail adoption of the stigmatized self-identity of someone who cannot cope with the pressures and demands of work. Within a medicalized discourse this reluctance to seek therapeutic intervention might be defined as an example of the way in which negative social stereotypes about mental health patients discourage potential patients from seeking help and thereby create 'unmet need'; however, it could also be argued that this represents a positive form of resistance to medicalization – a reassertion of resilience and selfhood in the face of an agency-robbing and self-diminishing therapeutic discourse. From exploring the dilemmas and ambivalence that characterize formal entry to the sick role we turned our attention to the experiences of those who receive 'treatment'.

The experience of treatment

Despite the apparent moral imperative against entering the sick role, several informants had eventually sought medical advice about coping with work stress, or symptoms. The decision to consult was not always driven by a conscious awareness of work stress; for instance, some informants consulted with physical health problems which their doctor then defined as a response to work stress.

The process by which the doctor acts as a mediator of work stress is discussed in the following section. This section concerns the way in which patients experience treatment and the way it influences their attitudes, beliefs and self-identity.

Informants reported several forms of treatment that they had received from their doctor, including the granting of sick leave for rest and recuperation, prescription of medication (commonly beta-blockers or antidepressants), and referral to a counsellor, psychotherapist, or other mental health specialist. The general practitioner was also valued as a 'sympathetic ear', capable of understanding the pressures of work and reinforcing the perceived link with health problems:

> . . . talking to my doctor has helped me a lot because I've explained to him, as I say, things like the work pressures, and he understood the sort of pressure I was under and I think that helps a bit to know that somebody else realizes what your pressures were and understands perhaps why you've had the trouble, the heart attack and that.

The type of informal support referred to above plays an important role in countering the stigma of consulting for problems relating to work stress. It reassures the patient that the decision to consult is a legitimate one, and that the doctor's time is not being wasted with something trivial. Choice of treatment was often negotiated between doctor and patient in response to the patient's concerns or preferences regarding, for example, medication:

> . . . he said, 'There are two ways of handling this. We can either give you some time off work, or I can give you some medication, something to take.' And I said I didn't want to take anything, so he signed me off work for a week. And he said, 'Come and see me in a week and we'll see how it goes.'

The element of patient choice, coupled with the sympathetic tone of the GP, may help to allay the patient's fears and anxieties about formally entering the sick role. It is as if the patient has to be slowly coaxed into adopting the identity of a 'work stress case' before the full gamut of therapeutic techniques can be deployed. When this process of identification has progressed, treatments which many informants were reluctant to countenance could be approached much more favourably, even when evidence of their efficacy was limited:

> Well I mean I could have felt a lot worse. This is what I said to her [the doctor] during the course of the time I was on Prozac. I might have felt dreadful if I was not taking it, but I didn't feel any better. It seemed to just keep the balance going. But it could have been worse if I hadn't taken it.

Fear of antidepressants appears to be twofold. First, there is concern that they might be physically addictive (actually unfounded), and secondly, there is a fear of adopting the identity of someone who cannot cope without them. Accepting a prescription for antidepressants is seen as a rite of passage into the stigmatized identity of 'mental health patient'; it signals, both to the patient and to others, an inability to manage one's mental life. This is not an identity that can be easily shaken off even after the patient has ceased taking the medication. He or she remains someone who once required medication for mental health problems. And the medical record is there to signal this information to potential future employers. Not surprisingly, this can generate reluctance to accept a prescription for antidepressants. However, once the first prescription has been issued and accepted a different set of imperatives shapes the patient's attitudes. First, the medication might work and lead to a genuine amelioration of symptoms, but, in any case, once the new identity of 'anti-depressant user' has been internalized, there is very little point to further resistance.

The same process appears to take place with counselling. Those who had not received counselling were often sceptical about its effectiveness, and reluctant to admit that they were the sort of person who would need such support:

> I know they might make you feel better but they can't sort the problem out. I am the only one who can sort the problem out.

> *So you said they can make you feel better, wouldn't that be useful?*

> No I wouldn't go to a counsellor because it would take two or three sessions for them to really understand what the problems are and by then I would probably have sorted it myself.

And again, from a different informant:

> *Would you consider going to anybody else, like a counsellor or somebody like that?*

> I can't honestly think what difference they could make, to be honest with you. I have got my counsellor sat there [points to husband], you know, we sit and talk and we air things out and we put the world to rights between us, we have a couple of drinks and watch a good film or I get on the phone and give my mum a ring and she is very depressing, my mother, so I listen to her for a bit and I feel better. I honestly can't think what they could tell me that would make it right.

As with antidepressants, those who had actually undergone counselling were much more optimistic about its efficacy:

> I think she helped me not to dwell on the depression so much but to see . . . I mean I felt totally lost. I had lost everything. I felt I couldn't do anything, that I was no good at anything. Being off sick allowed me to feel depressed which I never did before and initially I felt a lot worse than I did at work and it helped me to look at what I had achieved; that it wasn't all bad. She asked me what I'd managed to do since the last time and where perhaps I felt it wasn't very much she would say it was very good and things like that.

The public and scientific policy debate about the merits of counselling not unreasonably focuses on the question of whether or not it 'works'. The above evidence raises a more subtle series of questions. For the informant quoted above counselling appears to have helped ameliorate the symptoms of depression and low self-esteem. The perceived benefits came after a severe breakdown, where the patient had lost all ability to cope on her own. In these circumstances it seems that, up to a point, counselling can assist in the rebuilding of self-esteem (although it is important to recognize that the efficacy of counselling can only be properly tested by an extensive randomized controlled trial). From a pragmatic point of view it might be argued that effectiveness in ameliorating distress is the only important consideration, but we must also ask under what conditions counselling can work – to what question is counselling the answer?

We have argued that work stress is the phenomenal form taken by adverse experiences at work at this particular historical and cultural moment. It is a socially conditioned means of making sense of experiences which is shaped by political, economic and cultural changes. These changes create a tendency to experience problems at work within a medical–psychological frame of reference. Within this framework adverse experiences at work become embodied as negative emotional states and somatic symptoms. These emotional states and somatic symptoms may be shaped by discourse, but they are no less real for that. It is not the case that work stress does not exist, or that its physical and somatic correlates are a delusion; in the current historical and cultural context adverse experiences at work *really are* experienced as a threat to mental and physical well-being, at least by some people.

In this sense the discourse of work stress frames the question to which counselling, medication and other therapeutic techniques are the answer. However, rather than simply asking if these techniques 'work' we must ask what are the historical and cultural conditions of existence for the statement that 'counselling is the answer to work stress' to be true? If we have a heightened awareness of mental and physical frailty, a culture which celebrates victimhood, and an ever expanding therapeutic apparatus; if alternative frameworks for understanding and acting against problems at work have become ideologically and organizationally defunct, it is hardly surprising that the trials and tribulations of working life will be recognized as emotional problems (in a physiological as well as cognitive sense), or that therapies which 'treat' those symptoms by lifting the spirits or displacing negative modes of feeling should be experienced as a cure.

In this sense counselling can be compared with other responses to work stress mentioned by informants, such as smoking, drinking alcohol, having a massage, etc. It is a salve for low-esteem, a balm for hurt feelings. Seeking emotional support from others is also a key strategy for tackling negative modes of feeling. For many, these emotional comforts can be obtained informally from supportive family and friends. Only a cynic would dismiss the psychological benefits of talking through personal problems, discussing alternative solutions, being flattered, encouraged and affirmed by significant others. Counselling provides an ersatz intimacy; emotional support from people who are not emotionally involved. Where family and friends are unavailable or unsupportive, or where individuals are reluctant to burden people they are close to, or fear their disapproval, the counsellor can offer emotional support 'with no strings attached'.

The problem is that there *are* strings attached. It is precisely the formal detachment of the counsellor that marks the transition from informal emotional support to therapeutic intervention. Within limits, support from family and friends can be accommodated within prevailing norms of everyday emotional life and is unlikely radically to transform either self-identity or the social self (i.e. the self as perceived by others). Counselling on the other hand entails a very different form of social relationship; it entails formal recognition that the individual cannot manage his or her mental life without the active intervention of a therapist. Counsellors may be in the business of boosting self-esteem, developing coping skills and enabling their clients to act independently, but the very act of seeking 'professional help' may entail the adoption of a self-identity based upon low expectations of psychological resilience and mental competence. Counselling and other therapeutic interventions may 'work' in terms of ameliorating negative modes of feeling, but at the cost of a diminished self.

Our purpose here is not to assess whether antidepressants or counselling work, but to describe how they are experienced by the patient and the consequences that such treatment has for the patient's self-identity. We have noted that informants who had taken antidepressants or undergone counselling often appeared to be less critical of such methods than informants who had not been treated. It could be that attitudes towards treatment determine an individual's decision to consult, i.e. those who consult are already prepared to undergo treatment, and those who are sceptical about treatment do not consult. However, this does not fit well with the available evidence, because many of those who had received treatment described their initial reluctance to consult and an earlier scepticism about the efficacy of such treatment. It seems, then, that some patients undergo a reassessment of the treatment they are prescribed:

. . . at the time I remember writing a letter [to the doctor] that I didn't want counselling. It probably would have done me the world of good.

Why were you reluctant?

I was asked, but they seem to have counsellors for everything nowadays, and I suppose I thought it was all rubbish, but I don't think it was a load of rubbish. I think I should have probably seen someone.

You sound like you've had a change of heart about counselling.

Because I'm not depressed now. Whereas now I can look at it in a more sensible way, with a clearer mind, but when you're down in the dark emotionally you don't want anybody to help you. It's something that I think you have to just come out of eventually however long it takes.

In the above quotation the informant accounts for her change of heart about counselling by suggesting that her earlier reluctance was a symptom of depression. However, it could also be argued that the reappraisal of counselling is a consequence of adopting the self-identity of 'mental health patient'. An earlier reluctance to yield sovereignty over her mental life may have been eroded by the consultation process, as the patient comes to recognize herself as someone who is depressed and, therefore, in need of treatment. Once the new identity is firmly internalized, the earlier reluctance to undergo counselling can be rationalized from within the mental health paradigm as a symptom of depression. In this sense the therapeutic discourse of counselling and other interventions has an auto-referential mechanism for 'explaining' earlier doubts or resistances, in the same way that the devil can invoked by the convert to explain his or her earlier lack of faith.

In the light of Strong's criticism that early formulations of the medicalization thesis exaggerated both the practitioner's will to control and the extent of patient dependence, a degree of caution should be exercised in assessing the 'life-changing' character of counselling. Several informants who had received either counselling or medication reported relatively short periods of treatment, with a conscious strategy by their doctor or counsellor eventually to withdraw treatment and avoid dependence on clinical intervention. Moreover, we should avoid viewing the recipients of counselling as incapable of reclaiming sovereignty over their emotional life. Even so, for some informants withdrawal of treatment was only provisional and further treatment remained a possibility if symptoms recurred:

> . . . if something occurred, if some trauma came up, if the physical symptoms started to come back, I would go to him for medication.

It appears that for some work stress patients, although their exposure to treatment may be relatively short-lived, resort to clinical intervention may become normalized as the legitimate course of action to be taken when confronted by stressful events. This is closely tied to a lowering of expectations about one's personal resilience. The following quotation illustrates how undergoing treatment for work stress can make individuals conscious of the limits on their ability to cope with emotional demands:

> *Do you feel differently about yourself?*
>
> Yes. Yes. Yes. Definitely. You can't go on forever. You just can't cope with everything. You have a limit, and until you push the limit, you don't realize.

It should be borne in mind that this was a small qualitative study that can tell us little about the efficacy of the various treatments available for work stress, or the long-term consequences of medical intervention. However, the study does tell us something about the way in which people experience consultation and treatment for work stress. And there appears to be evidence that for some informants it entailed a transformative process in which initial reluctance to take up treatment options was slowly eroded. It is not an exaggeration to suggest that this transformation entails a reflexive reordering of the individual's self-identity, as the patient comes to think of himself as someone who is no longer competent to manage his mental life without the aid of therapeutic intervention. What role does the doctor play in this transformation?

The doctor as mediator of work stress

The factors affecting an informant's decision to seek medical advice have already been examined above. Severity of symptoms was a key factor; however, even where symptoms were very severe, the informant was not always conscious that problems at work were the main cause of the illness. Consultation with the doctor played an important role in making the connection between problems at work and symptoms of ill health in the individual:

> I didn't think about it being to do with stress. I just thought I was ill. You can only present the doctor with the physical symptoms. I wasn't particularly aware of any other problems.

Even where the patient already had a theory as to what was causing the symptoms, consultation with a doctor could lead to a reconceptualization of the problem in terms of work stress. For example, a nurse who suspected that her symptoms might be menopausal came to reassess the cause of her problems as a result of consultation:

> *And before you went to the doctor did you have any awareness that it might be to do with what was happening at work?*
>
> No. I think my brain must have probably blotted it out. I mean I'm not daft. I do know what the signs are but there is no way I thought that.
>
> *And when you went to see the doctor did she try to explore what the causes of the problems might be?*
>
> Yes. We did talk about work.
>
> *So it was during your discussion with the doctor that you became aware that it was work that was the problem.*
>
> Yes. I think I was thinking that my irritability and things like that, because I was getting hot flushes as well and I was putting it all down to perhaps being the onset of the menopause.

The point is not that symptoms are wrongly attributed to work stress (all of the informants reported problems at work) or that a monocausal theory is advanced for problems that have several causes (doctors often identify other stressful life events as well as work stress). The point is simply that the medical profession appears to play a key role in defining and reinforcing the perceived link between problems at work and symptoms in the patient. The immediate consequences for the patient may not be great, since the treatment for stress-related symptoms is likely to remain the same regardless of what is causing the stress. However, by defining work as a health problem the doctor's diagnosis is likely to have broader consequences for the patient. Usually, this influence is exercised indirectly, by granting sick leave and a diagnosis which the patient then takes to his or her employer, although, as the following quotation suggests, doctors may also be prepared to intervene directly in the relationship between employer and employee, in this instance during disciplinary proceedings:

> I explained what the situation was and he was kind enough to spend time compiling a letter to send to my employer to say that I was suffering stress. Because another one of the things that I was punished for, or at least they felt that I was guilty of, was the fact that one week I didn't use my car for work and I claimed mileage for using it. And then a week after I did use my car for work and I didn't claim mileage for using it and the doctor, I explained that to him and he said in his letter that I was suffering stress with my son [who was ill in hospital] and he understood that I would have been under a certain amount of stress during this period of time and, if they felt the need, they were quite at liberty to write to him and he would give them all the information.

Where the employer is a large company or organization with an occupational health department, a diagnosis of work stress can set in motion a series of formal procedures, for example:

> So I said: 'Oh I've brought a sick note in, and I've put a letter with it you see to explain that I've had two weeks off sick and I've got two weeks leave coming and after that I'm sure I'll feel a lot better and I had felt very pressurized at work recently.' That was the sentence that done it. And my boss rang me and said, 'Oh, I'm sorry, we can't actually let you come back.' And I said, 'Oh well, I'm fine. There's nothing wrong with me and the doctor has said I'm fine.' And he said, 'Yes but you've instigated (*sic*) that the Post Office is possibly to blame or accusations of whatever relating to your sickness; it's not as though you've had flu sort of thing or going blind or deaf or whatever', and I said 'Oh.' He said, 'Well, I'm afraid you'll have to see the Occupational Health Adviser and have a chat with her to see if she thinks you should continue.'

Whereas consultation with a doctor tended to be sympathetic and non-coercive, informants often felt that occupational health procedures were largely out of their control, and that they might be driven by the interests of the employer rather than those of the employee:

> I feel my illness was opportune for her [the manager], because she knew there were going to be ward closures by that time and it just meant there was one sister they didn't have to worry about.

The implementation of occupational health procedures not only meant that the employee/patient lost a degree of control over events, but often that the general practitioner was also obliged to fit in with the procedures, even if this went against his or her clinical judgement. For instance, in the following quotation an informant describes how she had to wait to see an occupational health doctor before being allowed back to work. Her doctor was obliged to provide her with sick notes for this period, even though he believed his patient was well:

> I had to wait weeks for this appointment, so I had to go back to the doctor's and say, 'Well, although you've said there's nothing wrong with me I can't go back to work because of this red tape', and so he just said, 'well I'll just give you sick notes.' He was quite understanding about it.

Several informants had eventually taken early retirement on medical grounds. Again, informants often reported that they felt that they had little control over the process that led to this outcome, and that they had effectively been obliged to retire. Several strategies were adopted by employers to persuade employees to take retirement on medical grounds, for instance offering the employee less attractive alternatives:

> ... she said that I could either return to my old job, at which stage there would be this [disciplinary] hearing, she could offer me a post two grades lower at a different hospital, I could be dismissed on grounds of ill health or I could look at early retirement. Well, I was just devastated. It had never occurred to me that I would do anything other than try and get back to work in my old job.

Alternatively, the employer might seek to smooth the passage to retirement by offering financial incentives, or by providing advice and support:

> ... they did send one gentleman towards the end who explained what retirement would mean and the tax and national insurance and how to apply it to the way you're going to live the rest of your life, all aspects of retiring. He came and talked to me and he was outstanding. He really was. They're very well trained and they're very good at that and they gave you a glossy folder of everything he said; lots of contact numbers including the Samaritans and all sorts of suggestions about what to do with your time and how to deal with things emotionally because they know they're not dealing with just old aged pensioners, lots of people have to take medical retirement. And they were brilliant. They really were.

The decision to take early retirement on medical grounds has significant consequences for employees/patients; at the least it means that they are likely to have difficulty returning to work at a later date, and at worst it might mean that they never work again. Despite the serious consequences that would ensue, the decision to take retirement on medical grounds was often taken by others, for instance the employee's GP:

> I told my doctor [about the symptoms] and he said 'No more Post Office – that is it.' And I argued and carried on but he said, 'No, no more Post Office. I forbid you to go back to the Post Office.' So that's why I left, because the doctor said. If I'd have said, Well I'm not going to, I'm going to stay, I'd have gone against his advice and he's a brilliant doctor and he was fantastic and he's known me since I was 15.

Note the way in which the status and prestige of the family doctor overrides the informant's perception of her best interests. On other occasions the decision not to allow the employee back to work was taken by the occupational health doctor, even if this contradicted the advice of the family doctor:

> *Was your doctor involved in your decision to take early retirement?*

> Not really. Not my doctor. The company doctor made the decision that he wouldn't allow me back to work [. . .] He [the GP] said the company doctor shouldn't have made that decision until he'd spoken to him because he reckons I am now probably 99 per cent fitter than most people at [company name] after what I had done but a decision was made and that was it.

Many informants found that their symptoms improved substantially after they had finished working; however, problems in adjusting to a new life without work were also reported:

> . . . after I left I got extremely depressed and despondent, total worthlessness. I wouldn't even think of trying to get a job because I wouldn't dream that I would even get an interview. I was absolutely, because I didn't want to give up the job. So I was angry. I still miss it.

Of course, only a small proportion of people who experience work stress will consult their doctor about symptoms relating to it, and even fewer will ultimately take early retirement on medical grounds because of those problems. But for many of those that do, it seems that there is an observable pathway, or career, leading from experiences in the workplace, through the identification of symptoms, the decision to consult a doctor, the definition of a causal link between work and ill health, the prescription of treatment, the issuing of a sick note, and the instigation of occupational health procedures that ultimately lead to retirement on health grounds. The doctor plays a key role in mediating this pathway, by formally defining the nature of the problem, establishing a causal link with experiences at work, and by directly or indirectly triggering the employer's response. Employees/patients often enter on this career with great reluctance, not just because of anxiety or scepticism about potential treatments, but often because they recognize that formally entering the sick role in this manner entails relinquishing the identity of someone who is capable of managing his or her own mental life without clinical intervention. In this sense, seeking medical help for work stress comes heavily freighted with negative moral sanctions, or stigma. It means becoming someone who lacks resilience when faced by the pressures of work, someone who cannot cope. Although the available treatments may (or may not) alleviate symptoms, they may also transform the self-identity of the patient, with consequences for resilience, at least in the short term. This is not so much an effect of the treatment, as of the decision that treatment is necessary. To adopt the self-identity of the 'work stress patient' is to be excluded from the group of mentally competent workers.

Once the new identity has been internalized many of the anxieties about treatment may evaporate, particularly where the doctor provides a 'sympathetic ear' and allows a wide degree of patient choice over treatment options. Many informants only occupied the work stress patient identity for a brief period of time. Their symptoms eased, either as a result of treatment, or because of changing circumstances at work, and they were unlikely to suffer long-term consequences, other than that they came to think of themselves as someone who had in the past, (and might in the future), required clinical intervention to help them cope with stress.

For a minority, the symptoms of work stress do not remit, and they go on to experience a process which is increasingly beyond their control, and which might ultimately result in the decision to take early retirement on medical grounds – a decision which is often heavily influenced, if not actually taken, by their doctor or employer. For such people (some of whom are relatively young) it is not an exaggeration to suggest that work stress has become the defining experience of their lives, effectively marking them as someone who cannot cope with the pressure of work, and severely limiting their future life chances.

Therapy or resistance?

The discourse of work stress is seductive. Western culture, particularly in Britain, is awash with incitements to infirmity: heightened awareness of mental and physical vulnerability; the rising moral status of the victim; and the proliferation of therapeutic apparatuses. These changes, coupled with the decline of alternative explanatory frameworks and oppositional strategies, provide an imperative towards the emergence of a relatively recent historical subject – the work stress victim. This new self-identity offers a ready-made framework for making sense of and responding to not just adverse experiences at work but their emotional and physiological correlates.

The response to problems at work depends largely on what people make of their experiences, and how they decide to react in response to them. However, people do not make sense of their experiences in isolation; rather they relate their personal experiences to a broader pattern of assumptions and expectations. This broader pattern can be referred to as the discourse of work stress, and it acts almost as a guide to behaviour or, at least, as a pre-existing framework within which experiences can be made sense of and decisions about future action can be taken. The discourse of work stress is an informal body of social knowledge. It comprises an accretion of lay experience, professional and academic opinion and media representations. Crucially, it reflects prevailing social and structural arrangements and is, therefore, historically specific.

As we discussed in Chapter 3, work stress is not entirely mediated at the level of consciousness or cognition. Over the broad sweep of the life course social experiences become written on the body in the form of unconscious emotional and physiological responses which can later be triggered independently of conscious appraisal. The physiological responses of the 'unconsciously knowing body' lend further credence to the belief that work stress is a universal, ahistorical, natural phenomenon. Unaware that these responses have been 'learned' over the life course, it is easy to assume that they represent a 'natural' limit on the body's capacity for endurance and resilience, further reinforcing the belief that work stress is fundamentally a biomedical response to the excessive demands and pressures of late capitalism. However, it is important to recognize that these 'symptoms' might be discursively constituted. A worker facing a high workload or job insecurity might not experience the symptoms of anxiety if he or she were confident that there were available strategies for addressing those problems, for instance trade union or political activity. Secondly, even if a physiological response was triggered by problems at work, the availability of alternative strategies might mean that they were interpreted differently by the worker; for example, sweating, increased heart rate and light headedness might be interpreted as anger and a spur to action, rather than as symptoms of anxiety and the prelude to illness.

Given these powerful social, cultural and physiological imperatives it is not surprising that so many workers come to experience problems at work as emotional/health issues. The identity of work stress victim not only offers a seemingly 'scientific' explanation of lived embodied experiences, it also offers a range of strategies for action: therapies and sick leave for some, exit from the workplace through early retirement on medical grounds for others, and for a few the opportunity to seek financial redress through the law courts. If these 'solutions' are so potent why is there widespread resistance to them? The answer to this question lies in the extent to which becoming a work stress victim entails relinquishing sovereignty over one's mental life. The ability to cope with stressful life events without recourse to therapeutic intervention has traditionally been viewed as a positive personal attribute, and those who have pushed themselves to the limits of psychological and physical endurance have been valued as 'high achievers'. The down side of valuing the ability to stand up to pressure is that those who fail to cope are stigmatized as weak or inadequate. Hence the reluctance among the informants to make the transition from being someone who is suffering work stress but coping with the pressure to someone who cannot cope without clinical support. The sharp distinction between 'copers' and 'non-copers' might be considered harsh, but it actually serves an important social function relating to human agency.

Agency, or the ability to engage actively with the world as a conscious actor, depends fundamentally upon mental competence. To be unable to cope with the demands of a stressful job and to seek medical advice is to relinquish one's identity as an autonomous social actor. For some this becomes inevitable; their symptoms are so acute and so debilitating that they are physically or mentally unable to carry on working. But for many others experiencing work stress, the choice of consulting a doctor or coping alone is not foreclosed; consultation remains something to be struggled against or lapsed into.

Of course, if those who currently struggle against the therapeutic imperative were to take up the treatments on offer their 'symptoms' might be ameliorated at least in the short term. And certainly the advocates of counselling and other mental health interventions would argue that treatment aims to restore impaired individuals to full mental competence. But what cannot be erased is the damage to self-identity caused by therapeutic intervention. Moreover, although blurring the distinction between copers and non-copers might reduce the stigma attached to consultation, this would also entail a lowering of expectations about human resilience. Rather than valuing the ability to cope with adverse circumstances, we would be valorizing human frailty and undermining agency.

Unpicking the threads of the work stress discourse to reveal its historical specificity and negative consequences for human agency does not imply that all is well with work. It may not be the pathogenic destroyer of health and well-being portrayed in the work stress discourse, but for many people the experience of paid employment is one of boredom, unfulfilled potential, frustration, uncertainty, dissatisfaction or alienation. One need not be a Marxist to recognize that the structural relationship between employer and employee is essentially antagonistic. Wage labour is founded on the worker relinquishing control over his or her productive activity in return for a wage. In the past this antagonism presented itself to experience in the form of political or trade union struggle. However, historical change has rendered this form of struggle ideologically and organizationally defunct – it no longer works as a way of making sense of experiences at work or as a practical strategy for pursuing workers' interests.

The work stress 'epidemic' has emerged in this political vacuum as the new phenomenal form of the antagonistic relationship between employer and employee. Adopting the subjectivity of the work stress victim is a way of making sense of adverse experiences at work and a guide to responding to them. We have argued that acceptance of this identity and the pursuit of therapeutic intervention entails a colonization of the worker's life world which is ultimately agency-robbing and conservative. Resistance to the therapeutic imperative is a form of heroism and should be applauded as such, but it should also be recognized that it operates within the parameters of the work stress discourse.

To reject the role of victim and decline therapeutic intervention does not in itself amount to a questioning of the fundamental assumptions of work stress, because it may still amount to having one's subjectivity structured within the terms of the discourse, but this time as a survivor/coper, i.e. as someone magically endowed with the personal qualities that the work stress victim apparently lacks. In terms of individual life experiences the latter subjectivity may be preferable to the former, but it actually reinforces the central claim of the work discourse, that the antagonisms of the workplace are best understood in terms of the ability or inability to remain mentally and physically healthy in the face of excessive demands and pressures. In either instance there is little challenge to the status quo.

A more active form of resistance can only come from stepping outside the work stress discourse and adopting a critical stance towards its assumptions, incitements, subjectivities and strategies. The most likely agent for this transformation is the mentally competent, emotionally resilient subject who has high expectations of human potential. Shaking off discursively constituted subjectivities, particularly when they are so deeply embedded in physiology, institutions and culture is more easily said than done. These identities are formed over the life course and take on a naturalized and immutable appearance. However, the historical specificity of the work stress phenomenon that we have attempted to disclose implies that it can be transitory, that more emancipatory modes of interpretation and opposition can be developed. Our aim has been to criticize work stress in theory; it can only be overthrown in practice.

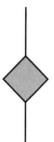

Appendix: methodology

Findings from two studies conducted by the authors are reported in the book. The first was a study of work and health among the adult population of the sea port of Dover in the South East of England. The second was a case study of occupational groups employed in general medical practice across the South East region. Both studies employed a similar research design – a postal questionnaire followed by in-depth interviews with a small number of respondents. The findings reported here are mainly from the qualitative components of the studies although some quantitative data from the Dover study is also included.

The Dover study

The postal survey

A 12-page questionnaire was compiled based on a pilot study of local ferry workers conducted in February 1997. Included in the questionnaire were a subset of the 'Short Form-36' instrument for measuring self-reported health status; the 12-item General Health Questionnaire which measures symptoms of minor psychiatric distress; a series of questions on help-seeking behaviour and health service uptake; questions on work-related stress and job insecurity; and other questions on personal details, employment status, health-related behaviour, and beliefs about unemployment. The survey commenced in September 1997 and was followed by two reminders to non-responders sent at monthly intervals. The data were entered into the Statistical Package for Social Scientists (SPSS); this process was completed by the end of January 1998.

The sampling frame comprised men and women aged between 16 years and retirement age (60 for women, 65 for men) who were registered with a general practitioner in the Dover locality of East Kent. The locality boundaries were defined by the East Kent Health Authority whose agency maintains the computerized register from which the sample was randomly selected (the computer software has a facility for random sampling). One in 18 of the sampling frame was selected, yielding 3101 names and addresses. It was suspected that migration and the recently deceased might inflate the register. To overcome this difficulty the sample was validated against the electoral register. There were 494 exclusions, giving a validated sample of 2607.

Of the validated sample 47 respondents (1.8 per cent) refused to complete the questionnaire and 1175 (45.1 per cent) failed to respond. This gave a response rate of 53.1 per cent (1385 cases). Given the modest response rate the demographic characteristics of respondents were compared with those of the sample and the population in order to assess response bias. Table A.1 lists several demographic variables and their distribution among respondents, the validated sample and the 1991 census population. It should be noted that the census data refer to residents of the Dover locality in 1991, whereas the respondent and sample groups exclude those living in the locality but not registered with a Dover GP and include those living outside the locality but registered with a Dover GP. Even so the census data provide a reasonable base-line for comparative purposes.

Table A.1 suggests that men and the 16–24 age band are under-represented in the respondent group although the difference is not great. Of greater concern is the under-representation of socially deprived respondents indicated by the car ownership and housing tenure variables. The data for the census population include pensioner households and it may be that

Table A.1 Composition of the respondent group compared with sample and census population by various demographic variables (all figures are percentages)

Demographic variables	Census population	Validated sample	Respondents
Gender:			
Male	50.3	50.5	47
Female	49.7	49.5	53
Age bands:			
16–24	18.6	16	13
25–44	44.5	46	42
45–65	37	38	45
Deprivation indicators:			
Rented accommodation	28.6 (all households)	Not available	20
No access to car or van	31.9 (all households)	Not available	14

those over retirement age are less likely to have access to a car. Even so, this apparent bias should be borne in mind when generalizing from the survey respondents to the population.

The follow-up interviews

The survey had asked respondents if they were willing to participate in a follow-up interview. A small number of informants was selected from the survey respondents who had indicated their willingness to be interviewed. Other information from the survey was also used in the selection process, namely reported levels of work stress, psychiatric distress (using the GHQ-12), and consulting behaviour. Twenty informants were selected, all of whom had reported high levels of work stress, although not all were GHQ cases and not all had consulted their GP about work stress. The interviews were conducted in the informants' homes. Duration varied but most were around one hour in length. An interview schedule was written in advance and modified over the course of the interviews. The interview schedule focused on key areas of interest, but the questions were open-ended to allow informants to introduce their own meanings and definitions. The interviews were tape recorded and transcribed verbatim. The data were analysed using the Atlas/ti computer program. Atlas allows for the development of theory that is grounded in the data. The process entails reading the transcripts through, developing a coding scheme for the emergent themes and developing a theoretical framework that charts the relationships between the themes. This is an iterative process which entails oscillation between the data and the theoretical framework with both being constantly revised. The data can then be sorted so that quotations relating to a particular theme can be grouped together. The findings are then written up with the inclusion of quotations from the interview transcripts that are illustrative of the key themes.

The case study of general medical practices

The findings reported here were derived from the second part of a two-stage research design. A postal survey provided a quantitative account of the prevalence of work stress in 81 randomly selected general medical practices across the National Health Service Executive South East region, using the indices for Karasek's job strain variables, Siegrist's effort–rewards model, and the GHQ-12 measure of psychiatric distress (among other variables). The quantitative findings are reported elsewhere; however, we were also interested in people's perceptions and experiences of work stress, and this required a qualitative methodology that would enable informants to express themselves in their own words. It was also considered important to examine the social relations and organizational dynamics of particular practices, rather than focusing on individual informants in isolation, and for this reason it was decided that whole practices would be selected for the follow-up study.

Site selection and recruitment of informants

When practices were selected for the postal survey they were also asked if they would be prepared to participate in the follow-up study. Those that refused to participate were obviously excluded from the selection procedure along with those that returned a response rate below 60 per cent. Practice profiles were produced for each of the remaining practices, comprising data on job strain and mental health status of staff (from the survey), and information on number of partners, geographical location and local population characteristics. The intention was to conduct interviews at five practices that appeared to have high rates of job strain and poor mental health, and five which had low job strain and good mental health. However, there were often inconsistent patterns in the distribution of variables and in the scores for different occupational groups in each practice, so the selection process was not as straightforward as had initially been envisaged. To overcome this difficulty each of the four researchers conducted an independent ranking exercise, identifying 10 'good' and 10 'bad' practices for follow-up, based on a subjective assessment of the information provided in the packs. The rankings were then compared at a group meeting where a final selection was made, based on which practices had been cited most often, and backed up by group discussion. As well as the job strain and mental health variables, practice size and geographical location were also considered in the selection of practices.

The selection procedure identified ranked lists of 9 'good' and 12 'bad' practices. The 'best' five and 'worst' five practices were then approached to see if the senior partner was still willing to participate in the follow-up study. All five of the good practices agreed to participate, but it proved more difficult to recruit from the list of 'bad' practices and only three of the top five could be persuaded to take part. Other practices from the list were then approached; the sixth practice refused to participate, but the seventh and eighth practices agreed.

The intention was to interview all staff willing to participate (within the occupational groups included in the survey), but some of the larger practices were reluctant to commit such a large amount of staff time given that it was not possible to reimburse costs. Recruitment was done via the practice managers, who approached staff and scheduled interview times. Each occupational group was adequately represented, although NHS Trust staff (district nurses and health visitors) were more difficult to recruit, and are therefore slightly under-represented. A total of 87 interviews were conducted, including 31 receptionists, 8 administrative staff, 10 practice managers, 9 practice nurses, 7 district nurses, 5 health visitors, and 17 doctors.

Data collection and analysis

Given the sensitivity of the research questions, it was felt that informants should be interviewed individually to ensure confidentiality and allow the informants to speak openly. A semi-structured interview schedule was used, focusing on the issues raised by the postal survey, and allowing digression where new themes were raised by the informant. The interviews took place at the practice, during work time. All of the interviews were conducted in private to ensure confidentiality. The informants were briefed to assure them that their comments would be entirely anonymous, and their permission was sought to tape record the interview. Interviews lasted from 20 minutes to an hour. The interview data were complemented by field notes detailing observations made about each practice.

All of the interview tapes were transcribed verbatim and analysed using the Atlas/ti computer package. The analysis deployed the iterative approach of grounded theory in which transcripts are read repeatedly to identify common themes. The themes were then used to develop a theoretical framework. The oscillation between data and theoretical framework was repeated several times, making modifications to the coding and the theoretical framework, until the best fit between the two had been achieved. The analysis was then written up, using illustrative quotations from the transcripts.

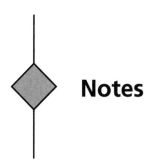

Notes

Preface

1 In the quotations from the qualitative interviews the following conventions have been used: '[. . .]' indicates that part of the transcript has been edited out; '. . .' indicates a pause.

Chapter 1

1 J.R. Jones, J.T. Hodgson, T.A. Clegg and R.C. Elliot (1998) *Self-reported Work-related Illness in 1995 – Results from a Household Survey*. Sudbury: HSE books.

2 J. Paige (1999) *Work Stress: A Suitable Case for a Code*. London: Trades Union Congress.

3 Health and Safety Executive (1995) *Stress at Work: A Guide for Employers*, HS(G)116. London: HMSO.

4 *Independent*, 6 July 1999, p. 6.

5 Unison (2000) *Stress at Work – A Guide for Safety Reps*. London: Unison.

6 J.H. Humphrey (1998) *Job Stress*. Boston, MA: Allyn and Bacon.

7 Ibid., p. 27.

8 J. Earnshaw and C.L. Cooper (1994) Employee stress litigation: the UK experience, *Work and Stress*, 8 (4): 287–95.

9 S. Kohler Moran, S.C. Wolff and J.E. Green (1995) Workers' compensation and occupational stress: gaining control, in: Lawrence R. Murphy *et al.* (eds) *Job Stress Interventions*. Washington, DC: American Psychological Association.

10 A.J. Grippa and D. Durbin (1986) Workers' compensation occupational disease claims, *National Council for Compensation Insurance Digest*, 1 (2): 15–23.

11 P.J. Rosch (1991) Is job stress America's leading health problem? A commentary. *Business Insights, School of Business Administration Journal*. Long Beach, CA: California State University.

12 L. Doyal (1979) *The Political Economy of Health*. London: Pluto Press.

13 The Committee on Safety and Health at Work. Presided over by Lord Robens, and reporting in July 1972.
14 Rt Hon. David Ennals in his introductory comment to *Stress at Work – MIND Report No. 3*. London: National Association for Mental Health (MIND), September 1971.
15 T. Cox (1993) *Stress Research and Stress Management: Putting Theory to Work*, Contract Research Report No. 61. Sudbury: HSE Books.
16 K. Parkes and T. Sparkes (1998) *Organizational Interventions to Reduce Work Stress – Are They Effective?* Oxford: Oxford University Press.
17 S.K. Parker, P.R. Jackson, C.A. Sprigg *et al.* (1998) *Organizational Interventions to Reduce the Impact of Poor Work Design*. Sudbury: HSE Books.
18 A. Smith (1999) Interim findings of the first British survey on the scale of occupational stress. Conference paper presented at 'Stress at Work' conference, London, 20 May.
19 Institute of Occupational Medicine (1999) *Evaluation of the Organisational Stress Health Audit*. Health and Safety Executive and Health Education Board for Scotland.
20 N. Simpson (2000) *The Effects of New Ways of Working on Employee Stress Levels*, Contract Research Report 259. Sudbury: HSE Books.
21 Health and Safety Executive (1998) *Managing Work-related Stress: A Guide for Managers and Teachers in Schools*. Sudbury: HSE Books.
22 Health and Safety Executive (1998) *Mental Well-being in the Workplace: A Resource Pack for Management Training and Development*. Sudbury: HSE Books.
23 Health and Safety Executive (1995) op. cit.
24 Ibid., p. 8.
25 J. Paige op. cit.
26 Health and Safety Commission (1999) *Management of Stress at Work*, DDE 10. Sudbury: HSE Books.
27 Health Directorate: Health and Safety Executive (June 2000) Discussion document, *Managing Stress at Work*, DDE 10. Summary of responses and actions. Available on-line at: http://www.hse.gov.uk/hthdir/noframes/stressdd.htm
28 Department of Trade and Industry (1998) *Fairness at Work*. London: The Stationery Office.
29 J. Lourie (1998) *Fairness at Work: Research Paper 98/99*, Cm 3968. London: House of Commons Library.
30 Department of Trade and Industry (1999) Good day for Britain's low paid, says Byers. Press release, 15 February, London.
31 Department of Trade and Industry (2001) National minimum wage. Available on-line at: http://www.dti.gov.uk/er/nmw/
32 Department of Trade and Industry (1998) op. cit.
33 Department of Health (1998) *Report of the Independent Inquiry into Inequalities in Health*. London: The Stationery Office.
34 Secretary of State for Health (July 1999) *Saving Lives: Our Healthier Nation*, CM 4386. London: The Stationery Office.
35 Department of Health (1999) Tessa Jowell launches the healthy workplace initiative. Press release, 9 March, available on-line at: http://www.ohn.gov.uk/ohn/school/workplace/release3.htm

36 London Hazard Centre (1999) *Hazards Campaign Charter: Health and Safety Demands on the Government*, 3rd edn. London Hazards Campaign. Available on-line at: http://www.lhc.org.uk/current/chtrhaz.htm

37 Quoted in R. O'Neill (1997) *Stress at Work: An October 1996 Conference Background Document*. Trades Union Congress. Available on-line at: http://www.tuc.org.uk/vbuilding/tuc/browse/browse.exe?1365&0&0&1&1, pp. 32–3.

38 Ibid.

39 *TUC Briefing on Occupational Stress*, 29 October 1996 (modified 2 July 1998). Available on-line at: http://www.tuc.org.uk/vbuilding/tuc/browse/browse.exe?348&0&0&1&1

40 Labour Research Department (1997) *Stress, Bullying and Violence – A Trade Union Action Guide*. London: LRD Publications.

41 Unison op. cit.

42 Transport and General Workers' Union (c.1998) *Safety Rep's Handbook – Some Key Health Issues*. Available on-line at: http://www.tgwu.org.uk/fea/srh/tng_h_srh_5.html

43 Institute of Directors (1998) *Health Matters in Business: Health at Work*. London: IoD.

44 J. Earnshaw and C. Cooper (1996) *Stress and Employer Liability*. London: Institute of Personnel and Development.

45 Confederation of British Industry (1999) *CBI Response to HSC Discussion Document 'Managing Stress at Work'*. London: CBI.

46 J. Earnshaw and C.L. Cooper (1994) op. cit.

47 R. O'Neill (1998) *Stress at Work: An October 1996 Conference Background Document*. Trades Union Congress. Available on-line at: http://www.tuc.org.uk vbuilding/tuc/browse/browse.exe?1365&0&0&1&1

48 *Daily Mail*, 6 July 1999, p. 1.

49 *Daily Express*, 6 July 1999, p. 16.

50 R. McKie in the *Observer*, 4 July 1999, p. 13.

51 S. Milne in the *Guardian*, 2 September 1999, p. 6.

52 R. Smithers in the *Guardian*, 9 September 1999.

53 *Daily Express* (1999) Lighten the load, Editorial, 6 July.

54 *Daily Mail* (1999) The compensation merry-go-round, Editorial, 6 July.

55 Department of Health (1998) *Report of the Independent Inquiry into Inequalities in Health*, p. 48. London: The Stationery Office.

56 Universities Safety Association and Universities and Colleges Employers Association (1999) *Dealing with Stress in Higher Education; How to Get Started: Management Guidance*, pp. 8–9. London: UCEA.

57 Labour Research Department (1997) *Stress, Bullying and Violence – A Trade Union Action Guide*. London: LRD Publications.

58 Universities Safety Association and Universities and Colleges Employers Association op. cit., p. 9.

59 Health and Safety Commission (1999) *Managing stress at work*. Discussion document. Sudbury: HSE Books.

60 Trades Union Congress (1999) *Stressing the Law*, TUC response to the Health and Safety Commission's Management of Stress at Work Discussion Document, p. 9. London: TUC.

61 Labour Research Department op. cit.

Chapter 2

1 W.B. Cannon (1925) *Bodily Changes in Pain, Hunger, Fear and Rage*. London: D. Appleton and Co.

2 W.B. Cannon ([1932] 1939) *The Wisdom of the Body*, second edition, revised and enlarged. New York, NY: Norton.

3 H. Selye (1936) A syndrome produced by diverse nocuous agents, *Nature*, 138: 32.

4 H. Selye (1946) The general adaptation syndrome and the diseases of adaptation, *Journal of Clinical Endocrinology*, 6: 117–230.

5 H. Selye (1950) *Stress*. Montreal: Acta.

6 H. Selye (1952) *The Story of the Adaptation Syndrome (Told in the Form of Informal Illustrated Lectures)*. Montreal: Acta.

7 H. Selye (1956) *The Stress of Life*. New York, NY: McGraw-Hill.

8 W.B. Cannon (1914) The interrelations of emotions as suggested by recent physiological researches, *American Journal of Psychology*, 25: 256–82.

9 H. Selye (1976) *Stress in Health and Disease*. Boston, MA: Butterworth.

10 T. Newton with J. Handy and S. Fineman (1995) *'Managing' Stress: Emotion and Power at Work*. London: Sage.

11 L.S. Hearnshaw (1987) *The Shaping of Modern Psychology*. London: Routledge and Kegan Paul.

12 C.R. Darwin (1859) *On the Origin of Species by Means of Natural Selection*. London: Murray.

13 C.R. Darwin (1872) *The Expression of Emotions in Man and Animals*, reprinted in 1979. London: Friedman.

14 G. Wallas (1914) *The Great Society: A Psychological Analysis*. London: Macmillan.

15 A. Flew (ed.) (1970) *Malthus: An Essay on the Principle of Population*. Harmondsworth: Penguin Books.

16 R.A. Peel (ed.) (1997) *Marie Stopes, Eugenics and the English Birth Control Movement: Proceedings of a Conference Organised by the Galton Institute, London, 1996*. London: Galton Institute.

17 H. Lee (1996) *Virginia Woolf*. London: Chatto and Windus.

18 W.B. Cannon (1925) op. cit.

19 W.B. Cannon ([1932] 1939) op. cit., pp. 226–7.

20 Although Cannon is often cited as the 'father of stress' he rarely used the term, preferring 'excitement' or 'emotional disturbance'.

21 W.B. Cannon (1925) op. cit., p. 269.

22 W.B. Cannon ([1932] 1939) op. cit.

23 G. Wallas (1914) *The Great Society: A Psychological Analysis*. London: Macmillan.

24 W.B. Cannon (1925) op. cit., p. 288, footnote.

25 W.B. Cannon ibid., p. 293.

26 F. Furedi (1994) *The New Ideology of Imperialism*. London: Pluto Press.

27 W.B. Cannon (1925) op. cit.

28 UNISON's Head of Legal Services, quoted in the *Independent*, 6 July 1999, p. 6.

29 R. Viner (1999) Putting stress in life: Hans Selye and the making of stress theory, *Social Studies of Science*, 29 (3): 391–410.

30 H. Selye (1952) op. cit.
31 H. Selye (1936) op. cit.
32 A. Patmore (1997) *Killing the Messenger: The Pathologising of the Stress Response*. Centre for Environmental and Risk Management, School of Environmental Sciences, University of East Anglia.
33 H. Selye (1956) op. cit., p. 4.
34 T. Newton with J. Handy and S. Fineman (1995) op. cit.
35 R. Viner (1999) op. cit.
36 R. Viner (1999) ibid.
37 T.J. Newton (1994) Discourse and agency: the example of personnel psychology and 'assessment centres', *Organization Studies*, 15 (6): 879–902.
38 R.D. Gillespie (1942) *Psychological Effects of War on Citizen and Soldier*. London: Chapman Hall.
39 R.S. Ellery (1945) *Psychiatric Aspects of Modern Warfare*. Melbourne: Reed and Harris.
40 I.L. Janis (1951) *Air War and Emotional Stress: Psychological Studies of Bombing and Civilian Defense*. Westport, CT: Greenwood Press.
41 N. Rose (1990) *Governing the Soul: The Shaping of the Private Self*. London: Routledge.
42 R.S. Lazarus, J. Deese and S.F. Osler (1952) The effects of psychological stress upon skilled performance, *Psychological Bulletin*, 49: 293–317.
43 OSS Assessment Staff (1948) *Assessment of Men*. Office of Strategic Services. New York, NY: Rinehart.
44 A.W. Melton (1947) *Apparatus Tests. Army Air Forces Aviation Research Programme, Research Report 4*. Washington, DC: US Government Printing Office.
45 R. Viner (1999) op. cit.
46 M.H. Appley and R.A. Trumbull (1986) *Dynamics of Stress: Physiological, Psychological and Social Perspectives*. London: Kluwer Academic/Plenum Publishers.
47 R. Viner (1999) op. cit.
48 R. Viner (1999) ibid., p. 401.
49 R. Viner (1999) ibid.
50 R.S. Lazarus, J. Deese and S.F. Osler (1952) The effects of psychological stress upon skilled performance, *Psychological Bulletin*, 49: 293–317.
51 R.S. Lazarus and C.W. Eriksen (1952) Effects of failure upon skilled performance, *Journal of Experimental Psychology*, 43: 100–5.
52 M.T. Matteson and J.M. Ivancevich (eds) (1987) *Controlling Work Stress: Effective Human Resource and Management Strategies*. San Francisco, CA: Jossey-Bass.
53 J.E. Hunter and F.L. Schmidt (1982) Fitting people to jobs: The impact of personnel selection on national productivity, in M.D. Dunette and E.A. Fleuschman (eds) *Human Performance and Productivity, Vol. 1: Human Capability Assessment*. Hillsdale, NJ: Erlbaum.
54 J.E. Driskell and E. Salas (eds) (1996) *Stress and Human Performance*. Mahwah, NJ: Lawrence Erlbaum Associates.
55 R.L. Kahn, D.M. Wolfe, R.P. Quinn, J.D. Snoek and R.A. Rosenthall (1964) *Organisational Stress: Studies on Role Conflict and Ambiguity*. New York, NY: Wiley.

56 S.E. Jackson and R.S. Schuler (1985) A meta-analysis and conceptual critique of research on role ambiguity and role conflict in work settings, *Organisational Behaviour and Human Decision Processes*, 36: 16–78.

57 K. Lewin (1952) *Field Theory in Social Science: Selected Theoretical Papers*, edited by D. Cartwright. London: Tavistock.

58 T. Newton with J. Handy and S. Fineman (1995) *'Managing' Stress: Emotion and Power at Work*. London: Sage.

59 D. Katz, N. Maccoby and N.C. Morse (1950) *Productivity, Supervision and Morale in an Office Situation*, Part 1. Ann Arbor, MI: Survey Research Centre, Institute for Social Research, University of Michigan.

60 B. Gardell (1971) Technology, alienation and mental health in the modern industrial environment, in L. Levi (ed.) *Society, Stress and Disease*, Vol. 1. London: Oxford University Press.

61 M. Frankenhauser and B. Gardell (1976) Underload and overload in working life: outline of a multidisciplinary approach, *Journal of Human Stress*, 2: 35–46.

62 G. Johansson, G. Aronsson and B.O. Lindstrom (1978) Social psychological and neuroendocrine stress reactions in highly mechanised work, *Ergonomics*, 21: 583–99.

63 R. Karasek and T. Theorell (1990) *Healthy Work: Stress, Productivity, and the Reconstruction of Working Life*. New York, NY: Basic Books.

64 B. Gustavsen (1988) Democratising occupational health: the Scandinavian experience of work reform. *International Journal of Health Services*, 18: 675–89.

65 T. Theorell (1993) On the end of the Swedish system, *Work and Stress*, 7: 201–2.

66 C. Eisdorfer (ed.) (1981) *Report of Committee to Study Research on Stress in Health and Disease of the National Research Council*. Washington, DC: National Academy Press.

67 M. Foucault (1980) *Power/Knowledge: Selected Interviews and Other Writings, 1972–1977*, edited by Colin Gordon, p. 118. Brighton: Harvester.

68 R. Porter (1999) *The Greatest Benefit to Mankind*. London: Fontana.

69 M. McKee (2000) Smoke and mirrors: clearing the air to expose the tactics of the tobacco industry, Editorial, *European Journal of Public Health*, 10 (3): 161–3.

70 J.T. Hodgson, J.R. Jones, R.C. Elliott and J. Osman (1993) *Self-reported Work-related Illness. Results from a Trailer Questionnaire on the 1990 Labour Force Survey in England and Wales*. Sudbury: HSE Books.

71 J.R. Jones, J.T. Hodgson and J. Osman (1995) *Self-reported Working Conditions in 1995: Results from a Household Survey*. Sudbury: HSE Books.

72 A. Smith, S. Johal, E. Wadsworth, G. Davey Smith and T. Peters (2000) *The Scale of Occupational Stress: The Bristol Stress and Health at Work Study*, Contract Research Report 265/2000. Sudbury: HSE Books.

73 I.C. McManus, B.C. Winder and D. Gordon (1999) Are UK doctors particularly stressed? *Lancet*, 354: 1358–9.

74 M.J. Burke, A.P. Brief and J.M. George (1993) The role of negative affectivity in understanding relations between self-reports of stressors and strains: a comment on the applied psychology literature, *Journal of Applied Psychology*, 78 (3): 402–12.

75 L.A. Clark and D. Watson (1991) General affective dispositions in physical and psychological health, in C.R. Snyder and D.R. Forsyth (eds) *Handbook of Social and Clinical Psychology*, pp. 221–45. New York, NY: Pergamon Press.

76 D. Watson and L.A. Clark (1984) Negative affectivity: the disposition to experience aversive emotional states, *Psychological Bulletin*, 96: 465–90.

77 D. Watson and J.W. Pennebaker (1989) Health complaints, stress and distress: exploring the central role of negative affectivity, *Psychological Review*, 96: 234–54.

78 R.A. Depue and S.M. Monroe (1986) Conceptualisation and measurement of human disorder in life stress research: the problem of chronic disturbance, *Psychological Bulletin*, 99: 36–51.

79 K.R. Parkes (1990) Coping, negative affectivity, and the work environment: additive and interactive predictors of mental health, *Journal of Applied Psychology*, 75 (4): 399–409.

80 R.D. Arvey, T.J. Bouchard, N.L. Segal and L.M. Abrahan (1989) Job satisfaction: environmental and genetic components, *Journal of Applied Psychology*, 74: 187–92.

81 L.J. Williams, M.B. Gavin and M.L. Williams (1996) Measurement and non-measurement processes with negative affectivity and employee attitudes, *Journal of Applied Psychology*, 81 (1): 88–101.

82 P.E. Spector, P.Y. Chen and B.J. O'Connell (2000) A longitudinal study of relations between job stressors and job strains while controlling for prior negative affectivity and strains, *Journal of Applied Psychology*, 85 (2): 211–18.

83 C.D. Spielberger, R.L. Gorsuch and R.E. Lushene (1970) *Manual for the State–Trait Anxiety Inventory*. Palo Ato, CA: Consulting Psychologists Press.

84 A. Smith *et al.* op. cit.

85 R. Karasek and T. Theorell (1990) *Healthy Work: Stress, Productivity and the Reconstruction of Working Life*. New York, NY: Basic Books.

86 J. Siegrist (1996) Adverse health effects of high effort/low reward conditions, *Journal of Occupational Psychology*, 1: 27–41.

87 H. Braverman (1974) *Labour and Monopoly Capital*. New York, NY: Monthly Review Press.

88 J.V. Johnson and E.M. Hall (1988) Job-strain, workplace social support and cardiovascular disease: a cross-sectional study of a random sample of the Swedish working population, *American Journal of Public Health*, 78: 1336–42.

89 M. Marmot, J. Siegrist, T. Theorell and A. Feeney (1999) Health and the psychosocial environment at work, in M. Marmot and R. Wilkinson (eds) *Social Determinants of Health*, pp. 105–31. Oxford: Oxford University Press.

90 R. Karasek and T. Theorell op. cit.

91 D. Goldberg and P. Williams (1991) *A User's Guide to the General Health Questionnaire*. Windsor: NFER-Nelson.

92 M. Calnan, D. Wainwright, M. Forsythe, B. Wall and S. Almond (2001) Mental health and stress in the workplace: the case of general practice in the UK, *Social Science and Medicine*, 52 (4): 499–507.

93 P.L. Schnall, K. Belkic, P. Landsbergis and D. Baker (eds)(2000) The workplace and cardiovascular disease, *Occupational Medicine: State of the Art Reviews*, 15 (1).

94 F. North, S.L. Syme, A. Feeney, J. Head, M.J. Shipley and M. Marmot (1993) Explaining socio-economic differences in sickness absence: the Whitehall II Study, *British Medical Journal*, 306: 361–6.

95 M.A. Hlatky, L.C. Lam, K.L. Lee *et al.* (1995) Job strain and the prevalence and outcome of coronary artery disease, *Circulation*, 92: 327–33.

96 P.L. Schnall, P.A. Landsbergis and D. Baker (1994) Job strain and cardiovascular disease, *Annual Review of Public Health*, 15: 381–411.

97 S.L. Sauter, J.J. Hurrell and C.L. Cooper (eds) (1989) *Job control and worker health*. Chichester: Wiley.

98 A. Steptoe and A. Appels (eds) (1989) *Stress, Personal Control and Health*. Chichester: Wiley.

99 M.G. Marmot, H. Bosma, H. Hemingway, E. Brunner and S. Stansfeld (1997) Contribution of job control and other risk factors to social variations in coronary heart disease incidence, *Lancet*: 350: 235–9.

100 S. Stansfeld, J. Head and M. Marmot (2000) *Work-related Factors and Ill Health: The Whitehall II Study*, Contract Research Report 266/2000. Sudbury: HSE Books.

101 H. Bosma, M.G. Marmot, H. Hemmingway *et al.* (1997) Low job control and the risk of coronary heart disease in the Whitehall II (prospective cohort) study, *British Medical Journal*, 314: 558–65.

102 J. Hallqvist, F. Diderichsen, T. Theorell *et al.* (1998) Is the effect of job strain on myocardial infarction due to interaction between high psychological demands and low decision latitude? Results from the Stockholm Heart Epidemiology Program (SHEEP), *Social Science and Medicine*, 46 (11): 1405–15.

103 J. Schwartz (2000) Imputation of job characteristics scores, in P.L. Schnall, K. Belkic, P. Landsbergis and D. Baker (eds) op. cit., pp. 172–5.

104 B.A. Greiner and N. Krause (2000) Expert-observer assessment of job characteristics, in P.L. Schnall, K. Belkic, P. Landsbergis and D. Baker (eds) op. cit., pp. 175–83.

105 S. Stansfeld, J. Head and M. Marmot op. cit., p. iv.

106 M. Marmot, J. Siegrist, T. Theorell and A. Feeney op. cit., pp. 105–31.

107 G. Davey Smith, M.J. Shipley and G. Rose (1990) Magnitude and causes of socioeconomic differentials in mortality: further evidence from the Whitehall Study, *Journal of Epidemiology and Community Health*, 44: 265–70.

108 R.G. Wilkinson (1996) *Unhealthy Societies: The Afflictions of Inequality*. London: Routledge.

109 Personal communication.

110 G. Davey Smith, M.J. Shipley and G. Rose (1990) op. cit.

111 G. Davey Smith, P. McCarron, M. Okasha and J. McEwen (2001) Social circumstances in childhood and cardiovascular disease mortality: prospective observational study of Glasgow University students, *Journal of Epidemiology and Community Health*, 55: 334–5.

112 G. Davey Smith, D. Gunnell and Y. Ben-Shlomo (2000) Life-course approaches to socio-economic differentials in cause-specific adult mortality, in D. Lean and G. Walt (eds) *Poverty, Inequality and Health*. Oxford: Oxford University Press.

113 J. Siegrist (2000) Work stress and beyond, *European Journal of Public Health*, 10 (3): 233–4.

114 J. Siegrist (1996) Adverse health effects of high effort/low reward conditions, *Journal of Occupational Psychology*, 1: 27–41.

115 S. Stansfeld, J. Head and M. Marmot op. cit.

116 M. Marmot, J. Siegrist, T. Theorell and A. Feeney op. cit., pp.105–31.

117 K. Sparks and C.L. Cooper (1999) Occupational differences in the work strain relationship: towards the use of situation-specific models, *Journal of Occupational and Organisational Psychology*, 72: 219–29.

118 J. Jonge, H. Bosma, D. Richard and J. Siegrist (2000) Job strain, effort–reward imbalance and employee well-being; a large cross-sectional study, *Social Science and Medicine*, 50: 1317–27.

119 M. Calnan, D. Wainwright and S. Almond (2000) Job strain, effort–reward imbalance and mental distress: a study of occupations in general practice, *Work and Stress*, 14 (4): 297–311.

120 J.M. Eakin and E. MacEachen (1998) Health and the social relations of work: a study of the health related experiences of employees in small workplaces, *Sociology of Health and Illness*, 20 (6): 896–914.

121 Ibid., p. 913.

122 R. Payne (1999) Stress at work: a conceptual framework, in Jenny Firth-Cozens and Roy Payne (eds) *Stress in Health Professionals: Psychological and Organisational Causes and Interventions*, pp. 3–16. Chichester: John Wiley.

123 R. Lazarus and S. Folkman (1984) *Stress, Appraisal and Coping*. New York, NY: Springer.

124 R. Payne op. cit., p. 8.

125 A. Bandura (1982) Self-efficacy mechanism in human agency, *American Psychologist*, 37: 122–47.

126 M. Friedman and R.H. Rosenman (1974) *Type A Behaviour and Your Heart*. London: Wildwood House.

127 C.D. Jenkins (1966) Components of the coronary prone behaviour pattern: their relation to silent myocardial infarction and blood lipids, *Journal of Chronic Disease*, 19: 599–609.

128 E. Riska (2000) The rise and fall of Type A man, *Social Science and Medicine*, 51: 1665–74.

129 D.W. Johnston, D.G. Cook and A.G. Shaper (1987) Type A behaviour and ischaemic heart disease in middle aged British men, *British Medical Journal*, 295: 86–9.

130 R.H. Rosenman (1996) Personality, behaviour patterns and heart disease, in C.L. Cooper (ed.) *Handbook of Stress, Medicine and Health*. Baton Roca, FL: CRC Press.

131 C.G. Helman (1987) Heart disease and the cultural construction of time – the type A behaviour pattern as a Western culture-bound syndrome, *Social Science and Medicine*, 25 (9): 969–79.

132 M. Whitehead (1995) Tackling inequalities: a review of policy initiatives, in M. Benzeval, K. Judge and M. Whitehead (eds) *Tackling Inequalities in Health: An Agenda for Action*. London: King's Fund.

133 C. Davison, G. Davey Smith and S. Frankel (1991) Lay epidemiology and the prevention paradox: the implications of coronary candidacy for health education, *Sociology of Health and Illness*, 13: 1–19.

134 J.B. Rotter (1966) Generalised expectancies for internal vs. internal control of reinforcement, *Psychological Monographs*, 80 (1): Whole No. 609.

135 P.K. Presson and V.A. Benassi (1996) Locus of control orientation and depressive symptomology: a meta-analysis, *Journal of Social Behaviour and Personality*, 11 (1): 201–12.

136 R. Perlow and L.L. Latham (1993) Relationship of client abuse with locus of control and gender: a longitudinal study, *Journal of Applied Psychology*, 78: 831–4.

137 P.E. Spector (1988) Development of the work locus of control scale, *Journal of Occupational Psychology*, 61: 335–40.

138 S.C. Kobassa (1982) The hardy personality: toward a social psychology of stress and health, in G.S. Sanders and J. Suls (eds) Social Psychology of Health and illness, pp. 3–32. Hillsdale, NJ: Lawrence Erlbaum.

139 A. Antonovsky (1979) *Health, Stress and Coping*. San Francisco, CA: Jossey-Bass.

140 S. Folkman and R.S. Lazarus (1988) The relationship between coping and emotion: implications for theory and research, *Social Science and Medicine*, 26: 309–17.

141 K.B. Matheny, D.W. Aycock, J.L. Pugh, W.L. Curlette and K.A.S. Canella (1986) Stress coping: a qualitative and quantitative synthesis with implications for treatment, *The Counselling Psychologist*, 14: 499–549.

142 D. Mechanic (1985) Some modes of adaptation: defense, in A. Monat and R.S. Lazarus (eds) Stress and Coping: An Anthology, 2nd edn., pp. 208–19. New York, NY: Columbia University.

143 R.S. Lazarus (1983) The costs and benefits of denial, in S. Bernitz (ed.) The Denial of Stress, pp. 1–30. New York, NY: International Universities Press.

144 J.E. Lynch (1977) *The Broken Heart: The Medical Consequences of Loneliness*. New York, NY: Basic Books.

145 L.F. Berkman and S.L. Syme (1979) Social networks, host resistance and mortality: a nine year follow up study of Alameda County residents, *American Journal of Epidemiology*, 109: 186–204.

146 D.C. Ganster and B. Victor (1988) The impact of social support on mental and physical health, *British Journal of Medical Psychology*, 61: 17–36.

147 S. Cohen and T.A. Wills (1985) Stress, social support and the buffering hypothesis, *Psychological Bulletin*, 98: 310–57.

148 Z. Soloman, M. Mikulincer and S.E. Hobfoll (1987) Objective versus subjective measurement of stress and social support: combat related reactions, *Journal of Consulting and Clinical Psychology*, 55: 577–83.

149 J.R.P. French Jr and R.L. Kahn (1962) A programmatic approach to studying the industrial environment and mental health, *Journal of Social Issues*, 18 (3): 1–47.

150 R.D. Caplan, S. Cobb, J.R.P. French, R.V. Van Harrison and S.R. Pinneau (1975) *Job Demands and Worker Health*. Washington, DC: US Department of Health, Education and Welfare.

151 J.R.P. French, R.D. Caplan and R. van Harrison (1982) *The Mechanisms of Job Stress and Strain*. New York, NY: Wiley.

152 G.E. Hardy and M. Barkham (1999) Psychotherapeutic interventions for work stress, in Jenny Firth-Cozens and Roy Payne, *Stress in Health Professionals:*

Psychological and Organisational Causes and Interventions, pp. 247–59. Chichester: Wiley.

153 R. Descartes ([1637] 1968) *Discourse on Method and The Meditations*, trans. F.E. Sutcliffe. Harmondsworth: Penguin.

154 R. Descartes ([1645] 1995) *Passions of the Soul*. Indianopolis: Hacett Publishing.

155 L.C. Bernard and E. Krupat (1994) *Health Psychology: Biopsychosocial Factors in Health and Illness*, p. 213. London: Harcourt Brace College Publishers.

156 J.W. Papez (1937) A proposed mechanism of emotion. *Archives of Neurology and Psychiatry*, 38: 725–43.

157 C.L. Sheridan and S.A. Radmacher (1992) *Health Psychology: Challenging the Biomedical Model*, p. 72. New York, NY: Wiley.

158 J. Siegrist (2000) Work stress and beyond, *European Journal of Public Health*, 10 (3): 233–4.

159 J. LeDoux (1996) *The Emotional Brain*. New York, NY: Simon and Schuster.

160 I.P. Pavlov (1927) *Conditioned Reflexes*. New York, NY: Dover.

161 J.P. Henry (1990) The arousal of emotions: hormones, behaviour and health, *Advances*, 6: 59–62.

162 J.W. Mason (1975) A historical view of the stress field, *Journal of Human Stress*, 1: 22–36.

163 R.M. Sapolsky (1993) Endocrinology alfresco: psychoendocrine studies of wild baboons, *Recent Progress in Hormone Research*, 48: 437–68.

164 R.M. Sapolsky (1994) *Why Zebras Don't Get Ulcers. A Guide to Stress, Stress Related Disease and Coping*. New York, NY: WH Freeman.

165 R.M. Sapolsky (1992) *Stress, the Aging Brain, and Mechanisms of Neuron Death*. Cambridge, MA: MIT Press.

166 M.J. Meaney, D.H. Aitken, C. van Berkel, S. Bhatnager and R.M. Sapolsky (1988) Effect of neonatal handling on age-related impairments associated with the hippocampus, *Science*, 239: 766–8.

167 H. Uno, R. Tarara, J.G. Else, M.A. Suleman and R.M. Sapolsky (1989) Hippocampal damage associated with prolonged fatal stress in primates, *Journal of Neuroscience*, 9: 1705–11.

168 R.M. Sapolsky (1991) Poverty's remains, *The Sciences*, 31: 8–10.

169 S. Cohen, D.A.J. Tyrell and A.P. Smith (1991) Psychological stress and susceptibility to the common cold, *New England Journal of Medicine*, 325: 606–12.

170 J.K. Kiecolt-Glaser, R. Glaser, E.C. Strain *et al.* (1986) Modulation of cellular immunity in medical students, *Journal of Behavioural Medicine*, 9: 311–20.

171 J.K. Kiecolt-Glaser and R. Glaser (1987) Psychosocial mediators of immune function, *Annals of Behavioural Medicine*, 9: 16–20.

172 J.K. Kiecolt-Glaser (1999) Stress, personal relationships and immune function: health implications, *Brain, Behaviour, and Immunity*, 13: 61–72.

173 W. McKinnon, C.S. Weisse, C.P. Reynolds, C.A. Bowles and A. Baum (1989) Chronic stress, leukocyte subpopulations, and humoral response to latent viruses, *Health Psychology*, 8: 389–402.

174 K. Vedhara, J.D. Fox and E.C.Y. Wang (1999) The measurement of stress-related immune dysfunction in psychoneuroimmunology, *Neuroscience and Biobehavioural Reviews*, 23: 699–715.

175 P. Martin (1997) *The Sickening Mind: Brain, Behaviour, Immunity and Disease*. London: Harper Collins.

176 A.A. Monjan and M.I. Collector (1977) Stress-induced modulation of the immune response, *Science*, 196: 307.

177 C.L. Sheridan and S.A. Radmacher (1992) *Health Psychology: Challenging the Bio-medical Model*. New York, NY: Wiley.

178 K. Bulloch (1981) Neuroendocrine-immune circuitry: pathways involved with the induction and persistence of humoral immunity, *Dissertation Abstracts International*, 41: 4447-B.

179 R. Ader and N. Cohen (1984) Behaviour and the immune system, in W.D. Gentry (ed.) *Handbook of Behavioural Medicine*. New York, NY: Guilford Press.

180 O.E. Brodde, G. Engel, D. Hoyer, K.D. Block and F. Weber (1981) The beta-adrenergic receptor in human lymphocytes – subclassification by the use of a new radioligund, *Life Sciences*, 29: 2189–98.

181 S.P. Galant, L. Durisetti, S. Underwood and P.A. Insel (1978) Beta adrenergic receptors on polymorphonuclear leukocytes: adrenergic therapy decreases receptor number, *New England Journal of Medicine*, 299: 933–6.

182 R. Ader, D.L. Felten and N. Cohen (eds) (1991) *Psychoneuroimmunology*. San Diego, CA: Academic Press.

183 J.S. Trilling (2000) Selections from current literature. Psychoneuroimmunology: validation of the bio-psychosocial model, *Family Practice*, 17: 90–3.

184 R. Ader and N. Cohen (1984) Behaviour and the immune system, in W.D. Gentry (ed.) *Handbook of Behavioural Medicine*. New York, NY: Guilford press.

185 J.M. Dwyer (1988) *The Body at War*. New York: New American Library.

186 R.H. Bonneau, P. Mormede, G.P. Vogler, G.E. McClearn and B.C. Jones (1998) A genetic basis for neuroendocrine-immune interactions, *Brain Behaviour and Immunity*, 12: 83–9.

187 R.L. Leriche, L. Herman and R. Fontaine (1931) Ligature de la coronaire gouche et fonction ches l'animal intact, *Comptes Rendus des Séances de la Société de Biologique et des ses Filiales*, 107: 545–6.

188 R.L. Leriche, R. Fontaine and J. Kunlin (1932) Contribution a l'etude des vaso-moteurs coronariens, *Comptes Rendus des Séances de la Société de Biologique et des ses Filiales*, 110: 299.

189 S. Wolf (2000) The environment–brain–heart connection: econeurocardiology, in P.L. Schnall, K. Belkic, P. Landsbergis and D. Baker (eds) op. cit., pp. 107–9.

190 B.H. Natelson (1985) Neurocardiology: An interdisciplinary area for the 80s, *Arch. Neurol.* 42: 178–84.

191 J.A. Armour and J.L. Ardell (1994) *Neurocardiology*. Oxford: Oxford University Press.

192 S. Wolf (2000) op. cit.

193 R.S. Eliot (1974) *Stress and the Heart*. Mt Kisco, NY: Futura.

194 K. Belkic (2000) Cardiac electrical stability and environmental stress, in P.L. Schnall, K. Belkic, P. Landsbergis and D. Baker (eds) op. cit., pp. 117–20.

195 K. Belkic (2000) ibid., pp. 117–20.

196 A. Steptoe and M. Marmot (2000) Atherogenesis, coagulation and stress mechanisms, in P.L. Schnall, K. Belkic, P. Landsbergis and D. Baker (eds) Ibid., pp. 136–8.

197 R.G. Wilkinson (1996) *Unhealthy Societies: The Afflictions of Inequality*. London: Routledge.

198 S. Wolf (1995) Discrete, patterned, and purposeful adaptive physiological adjustments integrated by forebrain influences, *Integrative Physiological and Behavioural Science*, 30: 190–200.

Chapter 3

1 J.M. Eakin and E. MacEachen (1998) Health and the social relations of work: a study of the health related experiences of employees in small workplaces, *Sociology of Health and Illness*, 20 (6): 896–914.

2 W. Wentworth and J. Ryan (eds) (1994) *Social Perspectives on Emotions*. Greenwich, CT: JAI Press Inc.

3 G. Bendelow and S.J. Williams (eds) (1998) *Emotions in Social Life*. London: Routledge.

4 S.J. Williams and G. Bendelow (1998) *The Lived Body: Sociological Themes, Embodied Issues*. London: Routledge.

5 P.E.S. Freund (1990) The expressive body: a common ground for the sociology of emotions and health and illness, *Sociology of Health and Illness*, 12 (4): 452–77.

6 B.S. Turner (1984) *The Body and Society*. Oxford: Basil Blackwell.

7 C. Shilling (1993) *The Body in Social Theory*. London: Sage.

8 P. Falk (1994) *The Consuming Body*. London: Sage.

9 E. Martin (1994) *Flexible Bodies*. Boston, MA: Beacon Press.

10 S. Nettleton and J. Watson (1998) *The Body in Everyday Life*. London: Routledge.

11 S.J. Williams and G. Bendelow op. cit.

12 S.J. Williams and G. Bendelow ibid., p. 3.

13 A.W. Frank (1991) For a sociology of the body: an analytical review, in M. Featherstone, M. Hepworth and B.S. Turner (eds) *The Body: Social Process and Cultural Theory*. London: Sage.

14 M. Merleau-Ponty (1962) *The Phenomenology of Perception*. London: Routledge and Kegan Paul.

15 M. Merleau-Ponty (1963) *The Primacy of Perception*. Evanston, IL: Northwestern University Press.

16 M. Merleau-Ponty (1965) *The Structure of Behaviour*. London: Methuen.

17 M. Merleau-Ponty (1968) *The Visible and the Invisible*. Evanston, IL: Northwestern University Press.

18 N. Crossley (1995) Merleau-Ponty, the elusive body and carnal sociology, *Body and Society*, 1 (1): 43–66.

19 S. Nettleton and J. Watson op. cit.

20 S.J. Williams (2001) Private communication.

21 A.W. Frank op. cit.

22 E.D. McCarthy (1989) Emotions are social things: an essay in the sociology of emotions, in D.D. Franks and E. Doyle McCarthy (eds) *The Sociology of Emotions: Original Essays and Research Papers*. Greenwich, CT: JAI Press Inc.

23 R. Harre (1991) *Physical Being: A Theory of Corporeal Psychology*. Oxford: Blackwell.

24 M. Foucault (1988) *Technologies of the Self*, edited by Luther H. Martin *et al*. London: Tavistock.

25 A. Giddens (1991) *Modernity and Self-Identity: Self and Society in the Late Modern Age.* Cambridge: Polity Press.
26 M. Maus ([1934] 1973) Techniques of the body, *Economy and Society*, 2: 70–88.
27 P.E.S. Freund (1988) Bringing society into the body: understanding socialised human nature, *Theory and Society*, 17: 839–64.
28 K. Marx ([1867] 1954) *Capital: A Critique of Political Economy*, Vol. 1, p. 80. London: Lawrence and Wishart.
29 J. LeDoux (1996) *The Emotional Brain: The Mysterious Underpinnings of Emotional Life.* New York, NY: Simon and Schuster.
30 K. Figlio (1987) The lost subject of medical sociology, in G. Scambler (ed.) *Sociological Theory and Medical Sociology*, pp. 77–109. New York, NY: Tavistock Publications.
31 P.E.S. Freund (1990) op. cit.
32 P.E.S. Freund ibid.
33 M. Barrett (1991) *The Politics of Truth: From Marx to Foucault*, p. 90. Cambridge: Polity Press.
34 L. Althusser ([1969] 1971) Ideology and ideological state apparatuses, in Louis Althusser, *Lenin and Philosophy and Other Essays.* London: New Left Books.
35 L. Althusser (1969) *For Marx.* Harmondsworth: Penguin Books.
36 L. Althusser ([1969] 1971) op. cit., pp. 162–3.
37 L. Althusser (1969) op. cit., p. 233.
38 R.W. Connell ([1979] 1982) A critique of the Althusserian approach to class (abridged from *Theory and Society*, 8 (3)) in A. Giddens and D. Held, *Classes, Power, and Conflict*, p. 146. Basingstoke: Macmillan.
39 M. Foucault (1980) *Power/Knowledge: Selected Interviews and Other Writings, 1972–1977*, ed. Colin Gordon. Brighton: Harvester.
40 M. Foucault (1980) *The History of Sexuality*, Vol. 1. New York, NY: Harvester.
41 M. Foucault (1988) op. cit.
42 M. Foucault (1988) *The Care of the Self.* New York, NY: Vintage.
43 A. Giddens (1987) *Social Theory and Modern Sociology*, p. 98. Cambridge: Polity Press.
44 M. Barrett (1991) op. cit., p. 89.
45 J.P. Sartre ([1943] 1969) *Being and Nothingness: An Essay on Phenomenological Ontology*, trans. Hazel E. Barnes. London: Methuen.
46 A. Giddens (1991) op. cit.
47 K. Marx ([1852] 1934) *The Eighteenth Brumaire of Louis Bonaparte.* London: Lawrence and Wishart.
48 S.J. Williams and G. Bendelow op. cit.
49 N. Crossley (1995) Body techniques, agency and intercorporeality: on Goffman's *Relations in Public, Sociology*, 29 (1): 133–50.
50 E. Goffman (1951) *The Presentation of the Self in Everyday Life.* New York, NY: Doubleday Anchor Books.
51 E. Goffman (1971) *Relations in Public: The Micro-Politics of Public Order.* London: Allen Lane.
52 E. Goffman (1967) *Interaction Ritual: Essays on Face-to-face Behaviour.* New York: Doubleday/Anchor Books.

53 E. Goffman ([1963] 1968) *Stigma: Notes on the Management of Spoiled Identity*. Harmondsworth: Penguin.

54 E. Goffman (1951) Symbols of class status, *British Journal of Sociology*, II: 294–304.

55 E. Goffman (1977) The arrangement between the sexes, *Theory and Society*, 4 (3): 301–31.

56 A. Hochschild (1979) Emotion work, feeling rules and social structure, *American Journal of Sociology*, 85: 551–75.

57 A. Hochschild (1983) *The Managed Heart: The Commercialisation of Human Feeling*. Berkley, CA: University of California Press.

58 A. Hochschild (1998) The sociology of emotion as a way of seeing, in G. Bendelow and S.J. Williams (eds) op. cit., pp. 3–15.

59 A. Hochschild (1979) op. cit., p. 569.

60 C. Wouters (1989) The sociology of emotions and flight attendants: Hochschild's *Managed Heart*, *Theory, Culture and Society*, 6 (1): 95–123.

61 S.C. Bolton (2001) Changing faces: nurses as emotional jugglers, *Sociology of Health and illness*, 23 (1): 85–100.

62 P.E.S. Freund (1990) op. cit., p. 469.

63 J. Lynch (1985) *The Language of the Heart*. New York, NY: Basic Books.

64 D. Kelly (1980) *Anxiety and Emotions*. Springfield, IL: Charles C. Thomas Publishers.

65 British Medical Association (1998) Second anniversary of BMA stress counselling service. Press release, 9 April.

66 C.S. Borrill, E.D. Wall, M.A. West *et al.* (1998) *Stress among Staff in NHS Trusts*. Sheffield: Institute of Work Psychology, University of Sheffield.

67 T.D. Wall, R.I. Bolden, C.S. Borrill *et al.* (1997) Minor psychiatric disorders in NHS Trust staff: occupational and gender differences, *British Journal of Psychiatry*, 171: 519–23.

68 C. Borrill and C. Haynes (1999) Health service managers, in J. Firth Cozens and R. Payne (eds) *Stress in Health Professionals: Psychological and Organisational Causes and Interventions*, pp. 105–18. Chichester: John Wiley.

69 M. Calnan and J. Gabe (1991) Recent developments in general practice, in J. Gabe, M. Calnan and M. Bury (eds) *Sociology of the Health Service*. London: Routledge.

70 D. Hannay, T. Usherwood and M. Platt (1992) Workload of general practitioners before and after the contract, *British Medical Journal*, 304: 615–18.

71 M. Calnan and R. Corney (1994) Changes in job satisfaction in general practice: a longitudinal analysis, *International Journal of Health Services*, 5 (2): 219–42.

72 V.J. Sutherland and C.L. Cooper (1992) Job stress, satisfaction and mental health among general practitioners before and after introduction of new contract, *British Medical Journal*, 304: 1545–8.

73 M. Calnan and S.J. Williams (1995) Challenges to professional autonomy in the United Kingdom? The perceptions of general practitioners, *International Journal of Health Services*, 25 (2): 219–41.

74 K. Appleton, A. House and A. Dowell (1998) A survey of job satisfaction, source of stress and psychological symptoms among GPs in Leeds, *British Journal of General Practice*, 48: 1059–63.

75 D. Hannay, T. Usherwood and M. Platt (1992) op. cit.

76 J. Howie and M. Porter (1999) Stress and interventions for stress in general practitioners, in J. Firth-Cozens and R. Payne, *Stress in Health Professionals: Psychological and Organisational Causes and Interventions*, pp. 163–76. Chichester: Wiley.

77 J. Firth-Cozens (1997) Predicting stress in general practitioners: ten year follow-up postal survey, *British Medical Journal*, 315: 34–5.

78 J. Firth-Cozens (1998) Individual and organisational predictors of depression in general practitioners, *British Journal of General Practice*, 48: 1647–51.

79 K. Appleton, A. House and A. Dowell op. cit.

80 M. Calnan, D. Wainwright, M. Forsythe, B. Wall and S. Almond (2001) Mental health and stress in the workplace: the case of general practice in the UK, *Social Science and Medicine*, 52: 499–507.

81 M. Calnan, D. Wainwright and S. Almond (2001 in press) Job strain, effort-reward imbalance and mental distress: a study of occupations in general medical practice, *Work and Stress*.

82 R. Karasek and T. Theorell (1990) *Healthy Work: Stress, Productivity, and the Reconstruction of Working Life*. New York, NY: Basic Books.

83 Ibid.

84 J. Siegrist (1996) Adverse health effects of high effort/low reward conditions, *Journal of Occupational Psychology*, 1: 27–41.

85 R. Karasek and T. Theorell op. cit.

86 J. Siegrist op. cit.

87 R. Lazarus and S. Folkman (1984) *Stress, Appraisal and Coping*. New York, NY: Springer.

88 J.M. Eakin and E. MacEachen op. cit.

89 P.E.S. Freund op. cit.

90 F.J. Buytendijk (1950) The phenomenological approach to the problem of feelings and emotions, in M.C. Reymert (ed.) *Feelings and Emotions: The Mooseheart Symposium in Cooperation with the University of Chicago*, pp. 127–41. New York, NY: McGraw Hill.

91 J. Siegrist op. cit.

92 D.D. Franks (1989) Power and role taking: a social behaviouralist's synthesis of Kemper's power and status model, in D.D. Franks and E.D. McCarthy (eds) *The Sociology of Emotions: Original Essays and Research Papers*, pp. 219–33. Greenwich, CT: JAI Press.

93 A. Hochschild (1979) Emotion work, feeling rules and social structure, *American Journal of Sociology*, 85: 551–75.

94 S.C. Bolton op. cit.

95 N. James (1992) Care = organisation + physical labour + emotional labour, *Sociology of Health and Illness*, 14 (4): 488–509.

96 M. Gothill and D. Armstrong (1999) Dr no-body: the construction of the doctor as an embodied subject in British general practice 1955–97, *Sociology of Health and Illness*, 21 (1): 1–12.

97 W. Yoels and J. Clair (1994) 'Never enough time': how medical residents manage a scarce resource, *Journal of Contemporary Ethnography*, 23: 185–213.

98 M. Foucault (1973) *The Birth of the Clinic: An Archaeology of Medical Perception*. New York, NY: Vintage.

99 P.S. Baker, W.C. Yoels and J.M. Clair (1996) Emotional expression during medical encounters: social dis-ease and the medical gaze, in V. James and J. Gabe (eds) *Health and the Sociology of Emotions*, pp. 173–99. Oxford: Blackwell.

100 A. Kleinman (1988) *The Illness Narratives*. New York, NY: Basic Books.

101 J.M. Eakin, E. MacEachen op. cit.

102 D. Wainwright and M. Calnan (2000) Rethinking the work stress 'epidemic', *European Journal of Public Health*, 10 (3): 231–3.

103 Z. Kmietowicz (2001) GPs shut surgeries in protest at government targets, *British Medical Journal*, 322: 1082.

104 P. Toynbee (2001) Doctors may protest, but they've never had it so good: the BMA cry out that their members are mistreated and overworked. *Guardian*, 2 May.

105 *Guardian* (2001) GPs present a host of complaints. Letters page, 7 May.

Chapter 4

1 J. Allen (1992) Post-industrialism and post-Fordism, in S. Hall, D. Held and T. McGrew (eds) *Modernity and its Futures*. Cambridge: Polity Press.

2 M. Castells (1996) *The Rise of Network Society*. Oxford: Blackwell.

3 U. Beck (2000) *The Brave New World of Work*. Cambridge: Polity Press.

4 R. Sennett (1998) *The Corrosion of Character: The Personal Consequences of Work in the New Capitalism*. London: W.W. Norton and Co.

5 *Guardian* (2000) Record payout for stressed teacher, 5 December.

6 *Guardian* (1999) Shock tactics, 13 November.

7 T. Bullimore (1998) *Saved: The Extraordinary Tale of Survival and Rescue in the Southern Ocean*. London: Warner.

8 F. Furedi (1997) *Culture of Fear: Risk-taking and the Morality of Low Expectation*. London: Cassell.

9 J.L. Nolan (1998) *The Therapeutic State*. New York, NY: New York University Press.

10 B.J. Burchell, D. Day, M. Hudson et al. (1999) *Job Insecurity and Work Intensification: Flexibility and the Changing Boundaries of Work*. York: YPS/Joseph Rowntree Foundation.

11 R. Sennett op. cit., p. 86.

12 A review of recent longitudinal controlled workplace closure studies can be found in J.E. Ferrie (1997) Labour market status, insecurity and health, *Journal of Health Psychology*, 2 (3): 373–97.

13 U. Beck (2000) *The Brave New World of Work*, pp. 76–7. Cambridge: Polity Press.

14 OECD (1997) Is job insecurity on the increase in OECD countries? *Employment Outlook*. Paris: OECD.

15 P. Gregg and J. Wadsworth (1999) Job Tenure, 1975–98, in Paul Gregg and Jonathan Wadsworth (eds) *The State of Working Britain*, pp. 109–26. Manchester: Manchester University Press.

16 F. Green (2000) It's been a hard day's night, but why? An exploration of work intensification in Britain. Public lecture given at the University of Kent, 23 June.

17 B.J. Burchell et al., op. cit.

18 F. Green op. cit., p. 14.

19 Ibid.

20 F. Green (2001) It's been a hard day's night: the concentration and intensification of work in late twentieth-century Britain, *British Journal of Industrial Relations*, 39 (1): 55–80.
21 Labour Force Survey (1992) *Quarterly Labour Force Survey*, Spring Quarter.
22 *Labour Market Trends*, June 1996.
23 F. Green (2001) op. cit.
24 S. Harkness (1999) Working 9–5?, in Paul Gregg and Jonathan Wadsworth, *The State of Working Britain*, pp. 90–108. Manchester: Manchester University Press.
25 F. Green (2001) op. cit.
26 J. Tomaney (1990) The reality of workplace flexibility, *Capital and Class*, 40 (Spring): 29–60.
27 T. Elger (1990) Technical innovation and work reorganization in British manufacturing in the 1980s: continuity, intensification or transformation? *Work, Employment and Society*, 4 (Special Issue, May): 67–102.
28 T. Nichols (1991) Labour intensification, work injuries and the measurement of percentage utilization of labour (PUL), *British Journal of Industrial Relations*, 29 (4): 569–601.
29 C.M. Campbell (1993) Do firms pay efficiency wages? Evidence with data at the firm level, *Journal of Labour Economics*, 11 (3): 442–70.
30 T. Nichols op. cit.
31 T. Nichols (1997) *The Sociology of Industrial Injury*. London: Mansell.
32 A. Bennett and S. Smith-Gavine (1987) The Percentage Utilization of Labour Index (PUL), in D. Bosworth and D. Heathfield (eds) *Working Below Capacity*, London: Macmillan.
33 D. Guest (1990) Have British workers been working harder in Thatcher's Britain? A reconsideration of the concept of effort, *British Journal of Industrial Relations*, 28 (3): 293–312.
34 B.J. Burchell *et al.*, op. cit.
35 D. Gallie, M. White, Y. Cheng and M. Tomlinson (1998) *Restructuring the Employment Relationship*. Oxford: Clarendon Press.
36 Industrial Relations Services (1996) Working harder, working longer: managers' attitudes to work revisited. *IRS Employment Review*, 600, January.
37 F. Green (2001) op. cit.
38 P. Waterson, C.W. Clegg, R. Bolden *et al.* (1999) The use and effectiveness of modern manufacturing processes: a survey of UK industry, *International Journal of Production Research*, 37: 2271–92.
39 N. Oliver (1991) The dynamics of just-in-time. *New Technology, Work and Employment*, 6 (1): 19–42.
40 G. Sewell and B. Wilkinson (1992) Someone to watch over me: surveillance, discipline and the just-in-time labour process, *Sociology*, 26: 271–89.
41 R. Delbridge, P. Turnbull and B. Wilkinson (1992) Pushing back the frontiers: management control under JIT/TQM factory regimes, *New Technology, Work and Employment*, 7 (2): 97–106.
42 C. Ichniowski, T.A. Kochan *et al.* (1996) What works at work: overview and assessment, *Industrial Relations*, 35 (3): 299–333.
43 H. Braverman (1974) *Labour and Monopoly Capitalism*. New York, NY: Basic Books.

44 R. Karasek and T. Theorell (1990) *Healthy Work: Stress, Productivity, and the Reconstruction of Working Life*. New York, NY: Basic Books.

45 R. Sennett op. cit., p. 99.

46 D. Marsh (1992) *The New Politics of British Trade Unionism: Union Power and the Thatcher Legacy*. London: Macmillan.

47 Cited in D. Marsh ibid., p. 11.

48 D. Marsh ibid.

49 N. Millward, A. Bryson and J. Forth (2000) *All Change at Work? British Employment Relations 1980–98, as Portrayed by the Workplace Industrial Relations Survey Series*, p. 20. London: Routledge.

50 D. Marsh op. cit.

51 N. Millward, A. Bryson and J. Forth op. cit.

52 Ibid., p. 220.

53 C.A.R. Crossland (1956) *The Future of Socialism*, p. 26. London: Cape.

54 C.A.R. Crossland (1956) ibid., p. 42.

55 C.A.R. Crossland (1956) ibid., pp. 32–3.

56 F. Fukuyama (1989) The end of history?, *National Interest*, 16: 3.

57 R. Hyman (1997) The future of employee representation, *British Journal of Industrial Relations*, 35 (3): 309–36.

58 D. Marsh op. cit.

59 Quoted in N. Bacon and J. Storey (1996) Individualism and collectivism and the changing role of trade unions, in P. Ackers, C. Smith and P. Smith, *The New Workplace and Trade Unionism: Critical Perspectives on Work and Organization*, Chapter 2, pp. 56–7. London: Routledge.

60 J. Kelly (1996) Union militancy and social partnership, in P. Ackers, C. Smith and P. Smith ibid., Chapter 2, pp. 41–76.

61 N. Millward, A. Bryson and J. Forth op. cit., p. 229.

62 D. Gallie, R. Penn and M. Rose (eds) (1996) *Trade Unionism in Recession*. Oxford: Oxford University Press.

63 F. Green (2000) Why has work effort become more intense? Conjectures and evidence about effort-biased technical change and other stories. UKC Studies in Economics. Canterbury: University of Kent.

64 A. Browne (2001) Antidote to the stiff upper lip: New Labour's best minds want to help you find your inner child, *Observer*, 21 January.

65 Antidote (2001) *The Antidote Manifesto: Developing an Emotionally Literate Society*. London: Antidote.

66 A. Samuels (2001) *Politics on the Couch: Citizenship and the Internal Life*. London: Profile Books.

67 J. Hewitt (1998) *The Myth of Self-Esteem; Finding Happiness and Solving Problems in America*. New York, NY: St. Martin's Press.

68 D. Summerfield (2001) The invention of post-traumatic stress disorder and the social usefulness of a psychiatric category, *British Medical Journal*, 322: 96.

69 R. Baggott (1998) *Health and Health Care in Britain*, 2nd edn. London: Macmillan.

70 M. Fitzpatrick (2001) *The Tyranny of Health: Doctors and the Regulation of Lifestyle*. London: Routledge.

71 *Guardian* (2001) Chemicals in hair dye could increase risk of cancer, 26 June, p. 7.

72 P. Skrabanek (2000) *False Premises, False Promises: Selected Writings of Petr Skrabanek*. Whithorn: Tarragon Press.

73 J. LeFanu (1999) *The Rise and Fall of Modern Medicine*. London: Little, Brown.

74 M. Fitzpatrick op. cit., pp. 27–8.

75 C. Davison, G. Davey Smith and S. Frankel (1991) Lay epidemiology and the prevention paradox: implications for coronary candidacy and health education, *Sociology of Health and Illness*, 13 (1): 1–19.

76 C. Davison, S. Frankel and G. Davey Smith (1992) The limits of lifestyle: reassessing 'fatalism' in the popular culture of illness prevention, *Social Science and Medicine*, 34 (6): 675–85.

77 American Psychiatric Association (1994) *Diagnostic and Statistical Manual of Mental Disorders*, 4th edn. (DSM IV). Washington, DC: APA.

78 S. Peele (1985) *The Meaning of Addiction*. San Francisco, CA: Jossey Bass.

79 F. Furedi (2002) *The State of Emotion*. Harmondsworth: Penguin.

80 D. Summerfield (2001) The invention of post-traumatic stress disorder and the social usefulness of a psychiatric category, *British Medical Journal*, 322: 95–8.

81 F.H. Norris (1992) Epidemiology of trauma: frequency and impact of different potentially traumatic events on different demographic groups, *Journal of Consulting and Clinical Psychology*, 60: 409–18.

82 *Guardian* (2001) Driver to get £500,000 after hitting girl, 16 February.

83 American Psychiatric Association (1994) *Diagnostic and Statistical Manual of Mental Disorders*, 4th edn. (DSM IV). Washington, DC: APA.

84 R. Coward (2001) Seeing is reliving: tragedies hurt us all, even if we are just watching on television, *Observer*, 4 March.

85 D. Summerfield (2001) op. cit.

86 *Guardian* (2000) Food bug trauma 'led to job loss', 4 May.

87 *Guardian* (2001) £330,000 for Hillsborough officer's late stress onset, 2 March.

88 *Guardian* (2001) Victims' groups angry over prison officers' payout: compensation culture comes under fire, 6 June.

89 G. Schelling, C. Stoll, H.P. Kapfhammer *et al.* (1999) The effect of stress doses of hydrocortisone during septic shock on post traumatic stress disorder and health related quality of life in survivors, *Critical Care Medicine*, 27: 2678–83.

90 S. Wessely, S. Rose and J. Bisson (2000) *A Systematic Review of Brief Psychological Interventions (Debriefing) for the Treatment of Immediate Trauma Related Symptoms and the Prevention of Post-traumatic Stress Disorder*. Oxford: The Cochrane Library, Update Software.

91 F. Furedi (2001) The silent ascendancy of therapeutic culture in Britain. Draft paper for Therapeutic Culture Conference, Boston, 31 March–1 April.

92 F. Furedi (2001) ibid., p. 2.

93 Guardian Unlimited (1999) Running scarred, March 24, available on-line at: www.guardian.co.uk/Archive/Article/0,4273,3843061,00.html

94 P. Rock (1990) *Helping Victims of Crime*. Oxford: Clarendon Press.

95 British Medical Association (1998) *Domestic Violence: A Health Care Issue?* London: BMA.

96 M. Fitzpatrick op. cit., p. 124.

97 D. Wainwright (1996) Empowerment unmasked: welfare professionals and the reluctant exercise of state power. Doctoral thesis, University of Kent: Thesis Collection.

98 F. Furedi (1997) op. cit.

99 R. Horrocks (1994) *Masculinity in Crisis: Myths, Fantasies and Realities*. London: Macmillan.

100 R.W. Connell (1995) *Masculinities*. Cambridge: Polity.

101 T. Newburn and E.A. Stanko (1995) *Just Boys Doing Business? Men, Masculinities and Crime*. London: Routledge.

102 I.M. Harris (1995) *Messages Men Hear: Constructing Masculinities*. London: Taylor and Francis.

103 A. Hobbs (1995) *Shattering the Myths of Masculinity. Health Lines*. London: Health Education Authority.

104 W. Kaminer (1993) *I'm Dysfunctional, You're Dysfunctional: The Recovery Movement and Other Self-Help Fashions*, p. 175. Reading, MA: Addison-Wesley.

105 P. Kramer (1994) *Listening to Prozac*. London: Fourth Estate.

106 S. Wessely (1996) The rise of counselling and the return of alienism, *British Medical Journal*, 313: 158–60.

107 M. Pringle and J. Laverty (1993) A counsellor in every practice?, *British Medical Journal*, 306: 2–3.

108 J. Eatcock (2000) Counselling in primary care: past, present and future, *British Journal of Guidance and Counselling*, 28 (2): 161.

109 F. Furedi (2001) op. cit., footnote p. 21.

110 F. Furedi (2001) ibid.

111 D. Wainwright (1996) The political transformation of the health inequalities debate, *Critical Social Policy*, 16 (4): 67–82.

112 F. Furedi (2001) op. cit., pp. 19–20.

113 K.J. Gergen (1990) Therapeutic professions and the diffusion of deficit, *Journal of Mind and Behaviour*, 11 (3–4): 359.

114 *Guardian* (2001) Vanishing calm: stress and mental health problems are showing a worrying rise in higher education, 12 June.

115 *Daily Telegraph* (1995) Counselling is offered for the death of a council, 25 October.

116 *Daily Telegraph* (1999) Taking the worry out of work, 6 April.

117 N. Rose (1990) Governing the Soul: The Shaping of the Private Self, p. 2. London: Routledge.

118 F. Engels (1958) *The Condition of the Working Class in England*, translated and edited by W.O. Henderson and W.H. Caloner. Oxford: Basil Blackwell.

119 R.E. Pahl (ed.) (1988) *On Work: Historical, Comparative and Theoretical Approaches*. Oxford: Basil Blackwell.

120 E. Hobsbawm (1975) *The Age of Capital 1848–1875*, pp. 219–20. London: Weidenfeld and Nicolson.

121 F. Furedi (2001) *Paranoid Parenting*. Harmondsworth: Penguin.

Chapter 5

1 R. Karasek and T. Theorell (1990) *Healthy Work: Stress, Productivity, and the Reconstruction of Working Life*. New York, NY: Basic Books.

2 R. Sennett (1998) The Corrosion of Character: The Personal Consequences of Work in the New Capitalism, p. 99. London: Norton.

3 *Guardian* (2001) Blair defies unions on reforms, 16 July.

4 A. Patmore (1997) *Killing the Messenger: The Pathologising of the Stress Response.* Centre for Environmental and Risk Management, University of East Anglia.

5 S. Wessely (1996) The rise of counselling and the return of alienism, *British Medical Journal*, 313: 158–60.

6 J. Eatcock (2000) Counselling in primary care: past, present and future, *British Journal of Guidance and Counselling*, 28 (2): 161.

7 A. Patmore (1997) op. cit.

8 I.K. Zola (1972) Medicine as an institution of social control, *Sociological Review*, 20 (4): 487–504.

9 I.K. Zola (1975) In the name of health and illness: on some socio-political consequences of medical influence, *Social Science and Medicine*, 9: 83–7.

10 E. Friedson (1970) *Profession of Medicine.* New York, NY: Dodds Mead.

11 A. Oakley (1980) *Women Confined; Towards a Sociology of Childbirth.* Oxford: Martin Robertson.

12 A. Oakley (1984) *The Captured Womb.* Oxford: Blackwell.

13 L. Doyal (1979) *The Political Economy of Health.* London: Pluto.

14 H. Graham and A. Oakley (1981) Competing ideologies of reproduction: medical and maternal perspectives on pregnancy, in H. Roberts (ed.) *Women, Health and Reproduction.* London: Routledge and Kegan Paul.

15 T. Scheff (1966) *Being Mentally Ill: A Sociological Theory.* Chicago, IL: Aldine.

16 M. Foucault (1965) *Madness and Civilization.* New York, NY: Random House.

17 H. Waitzkin (1983) *The Second Sickness: The Contradictions of Capitalist Health Care.* New York, NY: Free Press.

18 S.J. Williams and M. Calnan (1996) Modern medicine and the lay populace: theoretical perspectives and methodological issues, in S.J. Williams and M. Calnan (eds) *Modern Medicine: Lay Perspectives and Experiences.* London: UCL Press.

19 E.G. Mishler (1989) Critical perspectives on the bio-medical model, in P. Brown (ed.) *Perspectives in Medical Sociology.* Belmont, CA: Wadsworth.

20 K. Figlio (1977) The historiography of scientific medicine: an invitation to the human sciences, *Comparative Studies in Society and History*, 19: 265.

21 B.S. Turner (1987) *Medical Power and Social Knowledge.* London: Sage.

22 I. Illich (1975) *Medical Nemesis.* London: Calder and Boyars.

23 T. McKeown (1976) *The Role of Medicine.* London: Nuffield Provincial Hospital Trust.

24 A. Young (1980) The discourse on stress and the reproduction of conventional knowledge, *Social Science and Medicine*, 14B: 133–46.

25 P. Strong (1979) Sociological imperialism and the profession of medicine: a critical examination of the thesis of medical imperialism, *Social Science and Medicine*, 42 (12): 199–215.

26 S.J. Williams (2001) Sociological imperialism and the profession of medicine revisited: where are we now?, *Sociology of Health and Illness*, 23 (2): 135–58.

27 S.J. Williams and M. Calnan (1994) Perspectives on prevention: the views of general practitioners, *Sociology of Health and Illness*, 16 (3): 372–93.

28 M. Fitzpatrick (2001) *The Tyranny of Health: Doctors and the Regulation of Lifestyle*. London: Routledge.

29 M. Kelly and D. Field (1994) Comments on the rejection of the biomedical model in sociological discourse, *Medical Sociology News*, 19: 34–7.

30 P. Strong (1984) Viewpoint: the academic encirclement of medicine, *Sociology of Health and Illness*, 6 (3): 339–58.

31 S.J. Williams op. cit., p. 150.

32 R. Dingwall (1994) Litigation and the threat to medicine, in J. Gabe, D. Kelleher and G. Williams (eds) *Challenging Medicine*. London: Routledge.

33 U. Sharma (1996) Using complementary therapies: a challenge to orthodox medicine?, in S.J. Williams and M. Calnan (eds) *Modern Medicine: Lay Perspectives and Experiences*. London: UCL Press.

34 E. Annandale (1996) Working on the frontline: risk, culture and nursing in the new NHS, *Sociological Review*, 44: 416–51.

35 J. Gabe, D. Kelleher and G.H. Williams (eds) (1994) *Challenging Medicine*. London: Routledge.

36 M.A. Elston (1991) The politics of professional power: medicine in a changing health service, in J. Gabe, M. Calnan and M. Bury (eds) *The Sociology of the Health Service*. London: Routledge.

37 M. Haug (1973) *Deprofessionalization: An Alternative Hypothesis of the Future*, University of Keele Sociological Review Monograph, 20: 195–211.

38 J. McKinley and J. Arches (1985) Towards the proletarianization of physicians. *International Journal of Health Services*, 15: 161–95.

39 S.J. Williams and M. Calnan (1996) op. cit., p. 13.

40 H. Arksey (1998) *RSI and the Experts: The Construction of Medical Knowledge*. London: UCL Press.

41 D. Broom and R.V. Woodward (1996) Medicalisation reconsidered: toward a collaborative approach to care, *Sociology of Health and Illness*, 18 (3): 357–78.

42 M. Bury (1997) *Health and Illness in a Changing Society*. London: Routledge.

43 U. Beck (1992) *Risk Society: Towards a New Modernity*. London: Sage.

44 A. Giddens (1990) *The Consequences of Modernity*. Cambridge: Polity Press.

45 A. Giddens (1991) *Modernity and Self-Identity: Self and Society in the Late Modern Age*. Cambridge: Polity Press.

46 P. Conrad and J.W. Schneider (1980) Looking at levels of medicalisation: a comment on Strong's critique of the thesis of medical imperialism, *Social Science and Medicine*, 14: 75–9.

47 D. Armstrong (1995) The rise of surveillance medicine. *Sociology of Health and Illness*, 17 (3): 393–404.

48 D. Kelleher (1994) Self-help and their relationship to medicine, in J. Gabe, D. Kelleher and G. Williams (eds) *Challenging Medicine*. London: Routledge.

49 P. Conrad (1992) Medicalisation and social control, *Annual Review of Sociology*, 18: 209–32.

50 M. Foucault (1965) *Madness and Civilization*. New York, NY: Random House.

51 M. Foucault (1977) *Discipline and Punish: The Birth of the Prison*. London: Allen Lane.

52 M. Foucault (1973) *The Birth of the Clinic: An Archaeology of Medical Perception*. London: Tavistock.

53 D. Lupton (1997) Foucault and the medicalisation critique, in A. Peterson and R. Bunton (eds) *Foucault, Health and Medicine*, pp. 94–110. London: Routledge.

54 M. Foucault (1988) The political technology of individuals, in L.H. Martin, H. Gutman and P.H. Hutton (eds) *Technologies of the Self: A Seminar with Michel Foucault*, p. 146. London: Tavistock.

55 M. Foucault (1979) *The History of Sexuality, Vol. 1: An Introduction*. London: Allen Lane.

56 M. Foucault (1984) Space, knowledge and power, in P. Rabinow (ed.) *The Foucault Reader*. New York, NY: Pantheon.

57 D. Lupton (1997) op. cit., p. 99.

58 D. Armstrong (1994) Bodies of knowledge/knowledge of bodies, in C. Jones and R. Porter (eds) *Reassessing Foucault: Power, Medicine and the Body*, p. 25. London: Routledge.

59 R. Porter (1999) *The Greatest Benefit to Mankind*. London: Harper Collins.

60 C. Shilling (1991) Educating the body: physical capital and the production of social inequalities, *Sociology*, 25 (4): 653–72.

61 K. Malik (2000) Man, Beast and Zombie: What Science Can and Cannot Tell Us about Human Nature, p. 9. London: Weidenfeld and Nicolson.

62 S. Weinberg (1996) Reply, *New York Review of Books*, 3 October, pp. 55–6.

63 M. Bloor and J. MacIntosh (1990) Surveillance and concealment: a comparison of techniques of client resistance in therapeutic communities and health visiting, in S. Cunningham-Burley and N. McKeganey (eds) *Readings in Medical Sociology*. London: Routledge.

64 D. Lupton (1997) op. cit., p. 105.

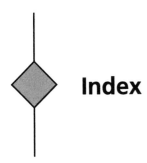

Index